Medical Editing

The Design of Books
Debbie Berne

The Chicago Guide to Fact-Checking
Brooke Borel

The Chicago Guide for Freelance Editors
Erin Brenner

The Craft of Science Writing
Siri Carpenter, editor

The Chicago Guide to Grammar, Usage, and Punctuation
Bryan A. Garner

What Editors Do
Peter Ginna, editor

Writing Science in Plain English
Anne E. Greene

The Craft of Scientific Communication
Joseph E. Harmon and Alan G. Gross

The Dissertation-to-Book Workbook
Katelyn E. Knox and Allison Van Deventer

Cite Right
Charles Lipson

Teaching and Mentoring Writers in the Sciences
Bethann Garramon Merkle and Stephen B. Heard

The Chicago Guide to Writing About Multivariate Analysis
Jane E. Miller

The Chicago Guide to Writing About Numbers
Jane E. Miller

The Chicago Guide to Communicating Science
Scott L. Montgomery

Developmental Editing
Scott Norton

The Subversive Copy Editor
Carol Fisher Saller

The Chicago Guide to Copyediting Fiction
Amy J. Schneider

Handbook for Science Public Information Officers
W. Matthew Shipman

A complete list of series titles is available on the University of Chicago Press website.

· BARBARA GASTEL ·

Medical Editing

A Guide to Learning the Craft and Building Your Career

The University of Chicago Press · Chicago and London

The University of Chicago Press, Chicago 60637
The University of Chicago Press, Ltd., London

Published 2025
Printed in the United States of America

34 33 32 31 30 29 28 27 26 25   1 2 3 4 5

ISBN-13: 978-0-226-82445-1 (cloth)
ISBN-13: 978-0-226-84492-3 (paper)
ISBN-13: 978-0-226-84491-6 (ebook)
DOI: https://doi.org/10.7208/chicago/9780226844916.001.0001

Library of Congress Cataloging-in-Publication Data

Names: Gastel, Barbara author
Title: Medical editing : a guide to learning the craft and building your career / Barbara Gastel.
Other titles: Chicago guides to writing, editing, and publishing
Description: Chicago ; London : The University of Chicago Press, 2025. | Series: Chicago guides to writing, editing, and publishing | Includes bibliographical references and index.
Identifiers: LCCN 2025015429 | ISBN 9780226824451 cloth | ISBN 9780226844923 paperback | ISBN 9780226844916 ebook
Subjects: LCSH: Medical literature—Editing
Classification: LCC R119 .G377 2025 | DDC 808.06/661—dc23/eng/20250725
LC record available at https://lccn.loc.gov/2025015429

♾ This paper meets the requirements of ANSI/NISO Z39.48-1992 (Permanence of Paper).

Authorized Representative for EU General Product Safety Regulation (GPSR) queries: **Easy Access System Europe**—Mustamäe tee 50, 10621 Tallinn, Estonia, gpsr.requests@easproject.com
Any other queries: https://press.uchicago.edu/press/contact.html

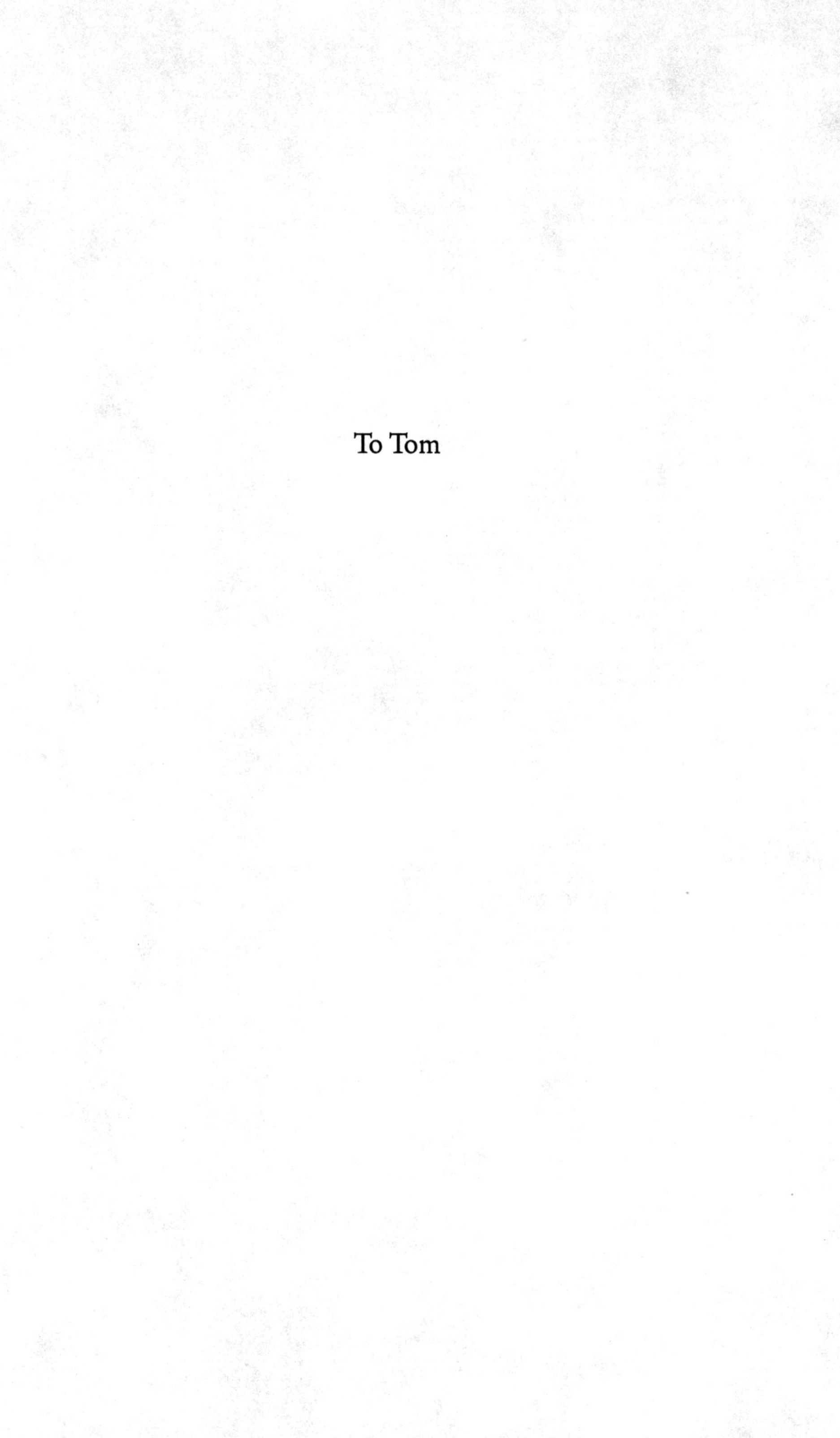

To Tom

Triage

BARBARA GASTEL (1993)

On its initial reading, this paper seems a mess.
(Or, to put it more politely, it rather lacks finesse.)
The punctuation's shaky, and the spelling's far from good;
If one tried to make it wordier, one doubtless hardly could.
The citations range in format, the tenses jump around.
Yet . . . it tells a tale, the research is hale, and the structure's fairly sound.
In short:
    It's got warts and halitosis and a very nasty zit,
    But a decent copy editor can help it quite a bit.

On its initial reading, this paper seems so-so;
And to be rather honest, it has a way to go.
Though the content and the prose style both are fairly strong,
Some key facts are missing, and in part the structure's wrong.
In the flow there are some problems, in the logic there's a catch,
And the abstract and the body do not seem to match.
In short:
    It needs some major surgery in order to survive.
    One hopes an author's editor shortly will arrive.

On its initial reading, this paper seems not bad;
It just would seem to benefit from polishing a tad.
But on more intense inspection, the paper comes up short:
The conclusions that are stated the results do not support.
The topic's not important; the approach is nothing new.
About very nearly nothing this paper's much ado.
In short:
    It lacks a heart; its lungs won't start; it has anencephaly.
    An editor of worth would not prolong its misery.

Contents

Preface . . . xiii

1. The Scope of Medical Editing . . . 1

Medical Editing as a Helping Profession . . . 2
The Five W's and an H of Medical Editing . . . 3
A Partnership with Authors, Readers, and More . . . 11
Key Points . . . 11

2. Key Resources for Medical Editors . . . 13

Style Manuals in Medicine and Related Realms . . . 13
Other Books . . . 18
Professional Organizations and Their Publications . . . 22
Educational Opportunities . . . 25
Online Resources . . . 28
Tools for Your Office . . . 31
Your Colleagues . . . 34
Key Points . . . 34

3. Approaching an Editing Project . . . 37

Understanding the Context: The Writing and Editing Processes . . . 37
Recognizing Differences Between Literary and Medical Editing . . . 48
Considering the Stage of the Manuscript—and of the Author . . . 49

Deciding on Levels of Editing . . . 52
Communicating About Expectations . . . 54
Determining What to Do in What Order . . . 56
Key Points . . . 57

4. Copyediting . . . 59
EDITING FOR MECHANICS AND MORE

Why Copyedit? . . . 59
Correcting and Querying . . . 60
Editing for Mechanics: General and Medical Aspects . . . 64
Editing for Conformity with a Publication's Style . . . 84
Editing Tables and Figures for Mechanics and Style . . . 88
Beyond Copyediting Per Se . . . 91
Key Points . . . 91
EXERCISE: *Some Sentences to Copyedit . . . 92*

5. Substantive Editing . . . 95
EDITING FOR CONTENT AND ORGANIZATION

Substantive Editing: Scope and Rationale . . . 96
Editing Journal Articles Reporting Research . . . 99
Editing Other Main Types of Journal Articles . . . 116
Using Guidelines for Journal Article Types . . . 121
Editing Medical Articles for General Readerships . . . 123
Editing Grant Proposals . . . 130
Key Points . . . 135
EXERCISE: *Organization of a Journal Article . . . 135*
EXERCISE: *Providing Substantive Feedback on an Abstract . . . 137*

6. Editing Conference and Career Communications . . . 139

Editing Conference Communications: Presentations and More . . . 139
Editing Career-Related Communications . . . 149
Key Points . . . 158

7. Additional Aspects of Medical Manuscript Editing . . . 159

Editing for Conciseness . . . 159
Editing for Readability . . . 162
Editing Writing by and for Non-Native Users of English . . . 165
Proofreading: A Related Skill . . . 170
Avoiding Overediting and Other Pitfalls . . . 173

Working Effectively with Authors: The Author-Editor Relationship ... 175
Key Points ... 184
EXERCISE: *Editing for Conciseness* ... 185

8. Ethics ... 187
YOUR OWN AND OTHERS'

Underlying Principles ... 187
Ethical Obligations of Medical Editors ... 189
Editors as Resources Regarding Medical Authors' Ethics ... 191
Approaching Ethical Issues ... 197
Key Points ... 198
EXERCISE: *Cases to Consider* ... 199

9. Careers in Medical Editing ... 203

Medical Editing: The Range of Substance and Settings ... 203
Seeking and Pursuing Medical Editing Positions ... 208
Taking Medical Editing Tests for Employment ... 217
Certificates and Certifications ... 218
Considerations for Freelance Medical Editors ... 221
Working Remotely ... 224
Continuing to Develop as a Medical Editor ... 226
Maintaining Motivation ... 227
Satisfactions of Medical Editing ... 230
Key Points ... 230

Acknowledgments ... 233

APPENDIX 1
Creating and Using a Style Sheet for an Abstract ... 235

APPENDIX 2
A Style Sheet for an Article for General Readers ... 239

Answer Keys: Exercises ... 241
List of Abbreviations ... 253
Glossary ... 255
References ... 261
Index ... 267

Preface

If you picked up this book, quite likely you are thinking of becoming a medical editor and wish to know more about the field. Perhaps you are a new medical editor seeking more background, especially in areas that distinguish medical from other editing. Or maybe you are more established and want materials on medical editing for those you mentor. I have been in all three situations, and the current book provides guidance of types I would have welcomed at various times in my medical editing journey.

The origins of this book date back many years, at least to my medical education. In middle school, high school, and college, I edited student publications while dividing my studies between sciences and humanities. I debated seeking a career in communicating science or medicine. However, clear paths to such careers were lacking at the time. Therefore, I opted to take the "easy" way out and attend medical school.

Early in my medical education, a fellow student noted that a journal based at our medical school was seeking student assistant editors. I applied and was thrilled to be accepted. That journal became my medical school home. While classmates reveled at being invited late at night to scrub in on a surgery or work up a fever, I lost track of time until all hours editing scientific papers. Medical editing, I found, combined my love of medical content and my penchant for the craft of communication. I realized that it was the place for me.

Thus, after much reflection, I decided to seek a career in medical communication rather than clinical medicine. I spent my remaining medical school elective time obtaining a master's degree in public health, knowing that a background in epidemiology, biostatistics, and related subjects would aid me as a medical writer and editor. Meanwhile, I continued serving the medical journal and did editing for the school of public health.

After medical school graduation, I continued my learning with an American Association for the Advancement of Science mass media fellowship at *Newsweek* magazine. An editorial skill I learned and extensively used there was fact-checking. I then obtained positions at the National Institutes of Health and the National Center for Health Care Technology; doing a mix of writing, editing, and administration, I continued learning about medicine, communication, and more. My time at *Newsweek* and then in government was in essence a residency in medical editing and related realms.

In keeping with my liking of communication, I had enjoyed being a teaching assistant during summers back home during medical school. So, when a position teaching science writing opened up, I applied for it. To my surprise, I was accepted. Teaching, I thought, could be interesting to try for a couple of years. But I am still teaching many years later. One of my favorite subjects to teach is medical editing. I also find that teaching—and especially giving feedback on student writing—draws on some of the same skills as editing. And my faculty position is a fine base for editorial work. My editing while a faculty member has included editing biomedical journal articles for colleagues and others, editing conference proceedings, and serving as editor-in-chief of *Science Editor*, the periodical of the Council of Science Editors.

Along the way, I spent two years teaching scientific writing at what is now Peking University Health Center and doing English-language editing for journals published by the Chinese Medical Association. The experience deepened my longstanding interest in international communication of medical research, and it helped me learn about editing medical writing by international authors and for international readers. It eventually led to my directing the US aspect of a program to train medical editors in China and elsewhere in Asia and hosting editorial interns from the program. In turn, those experiences led to major roles in establishing and leading AuthorAID, an international program largely to help researchers in low- and middle-income countries to write about and publish their work.

For most of my career, I have been at Texas A&M University, where I direct the graduate program in science and technology journalism (largely a professional program in science writing and science editing). My teaching in this program includes courses in science editing, with an emphasis on medical editing; often the students do editorial internships, and often they pursue careers in medical or other editing. In addition, I teach in the University of Chicago certificate program in medical writing and editing, for which I developed and deliver the course Fundamentals of Substantive Editing and Publication Ethics.

The current book is largely an outgrowth of teaching I have done at Texas A&M University and for the University of Chicago program. It is intended primarily to introduce the field of medical editing, to aid in developing core knowledge and skills in this field, and to help in exploring career possibilities in it. As well as presenting editorial basics as applied to medical editing, the book addresses topics specific to this field—for example, norms for medical writing and editing, including those for distinctive types of journal articles; ways that editors can efficiently and effectively brief themselves on medical terminology and content; ethical obligations inherent in editing medical content; and the range of employment available in medical editing. Throughout, the book also emphasizes resources on medical editing and for medical editors.

This book is targeted mainly to prospective and early-career medical editors. More experienced medical editors also may find some of the content useful, as may individuals in related fields and general editors tasked with editing an occasional medical piece. In addition, teachers of related subjects, such as medical writing or technical editing, may find this book helpful to consult when developing parts of their courses. Similarly, supervisors may find the book useful in mentoring interns or new hires.

Different readers can approach this book in different ways. For instance, a prospective or beginning medical editor may well read the book from cover to cover. A medical copyeditor seeking to enter substantive medical editing may focus mainly on the chapter on that subject. A job seeker might read the last chapter (on medical editing careers) first. Established medical editors might skim the book, zeroing in on tips and resources they have not yet encountered and perhaps comparing their perspectives with those presented. Teachers, trainers, and supervisors may draw on the book for content to share. Accordingly, each chapter is designed to be freestanding, even if slight redundancy therefore results. Because resources for medical editors serve as a foundation for work in the field, the chapter on resources appears early in the book, rather than near the end as is common. The book also is designed to be information-rich yet easy to skim and quick to read.

Given the wide scope of medical editing, this book cannot address every variety in depth. Rather, in addition to addressing general aspects, it focuses most on editing journal submissions, articles for general readerships, grant proposals, and oral and poster presentations. Those who will edit other types of medical writing—such as regulatory documents, continuing medical education (CME) products, marketing and advertising materials, and patient-education resources—can apply many basics from this book, use approaches in it as models, and learn specifics from resources on such types of communications and from mentors specializing in these realms.

Medical editing is a dynamic field. Resources, tools, procedures, and norms in it change over time, and so some specifics in this book will become out of date. The core guidance in this book, however, is likely to endure, especially because the book emphasizes approaches rather than rules. And this book, which includes advice on staying current, can serve as a foundation for continued learning as the field continues to evolve.

As this book goes to press, the aspect of medical editing that seems to be evolving fastest, and about which medical editors seem to vary most in views and practice, is the use of electronic tools, especially artificial intelligence (AI). Therefore, after much reflection and discussion, the decision was reached not to try to present many specifics in this regard. However, resources and approaches noted in this book can help readers keep up in this realm. Likewise, over the years the foundation this book provides in medical editing can help readers decide which such tools to use, what to use them for, and how to use them—and to validly assess and apply their output.

This book is written primarily from a US standpoint, and it focuses on English-language medical editing. But especially given my international experiences and interests, I have tried to make much of it applicable as well to medical editing in other countries, cultures, and languages and to write in a way easy for international readers to understand. I hope that much of this book can aid prospective and current medical editors regardless of country and that international peers will adapt parts of the content as warranted when guiding those who are less experienced.

In the pages that follow, I hope to share my enthusiasm for medical editing as a craft and a career and to facilitate others' forays in this field. May your journey in medical editing be as rewarding as mine.

· 1 ·

The Scope of Medical Editing

I am lucky to know many fine medical editors. Nearly all share an interest in medicine, a love of language, and a commitment to excellence. But in other ways, the editors vary greatly. Some have degrees in the liberal arts, some in the sciences, and some in other fields. Some have advanced degrees, others not. Some are trained as health professionals. Some work at medical journals, health science centers, corporations, or other institutions; others freelance full-time. Some focus on editing journal articles, grant proposals, materials for general readerships, or other items; others edit a mix. Some are relatively quiet, others quite outgoing.

The scope of work performed by these medical editors also varies widely. As well as dealing with grammar, punctuation, and other mechanics, it commonly includes attention to required style and format. It may strive to increase readability. It may address organization, logic, and other substantive aspects. It often requires flexibility and judgment, an understanding of writers and readers, and—given medical editors' interaction with authors and others—good interpersonal skills. In short, there is little reality to the stereotype of a medical editor grimly correcting the grammar of a journal article.

Accordingly, this chapter offers an overview of the scope of medical editing. In doing so, it provides a foundation for the rest of the book.

Medical Editing as a Helping Profession

Medical information can be a matter of life and death. Health professionals need it to serve patients. Researchers need it as a foundation for advancing medical knowledge. Members of the public need it to safeguard their health. To serve these functions, medical writing must contain information that is correct and complete. The writing also must be clear, lest it be misinterpreted. The material also should be written readably, and perhaps engagingly, to help ensure that it will indeed be read. Medical editors help ensure that medical writing succeeds in all these regards.

Also, to succeed professionally, many people must write well about medical matters. To obtain funding to conduct their investigations, researchers must write grant proposals that are clear and persuasive. Upon completing the research, they need to write articles that peer reviewers and journal editors will deem publishable. Physicians and other health professionals may want or need to write patient information materials, book chapters, and other items. Professional writers must ensure that their medical writings meet appropriate standards. Even the best writers benefit from the input of an editor. Editors can help authors from all these professions communicate well and achieve their career goals.

Publishers seek to offer writing that contains sound information, communicates it effectively, is sufficiently polished, and meets high standards in other respects (for example, regarding copyright compliance). Publishers also often require that writing follows a given style and format. In addition, they may want the writing to be concise, both to conserve resources such as paper and because of readers' limited time and attention spans. By helping to ensure that materials meet publishers' expectations, medical editors help publishers to attain their objectives and achieve or maintain favorable reputations.

In short, medical editors serve readers, authors, and publishers. They thus serve public well-being and help others do so. Medical editing is therefore a helping profession. Indeed, some editors prefer medical editing because of the chance to contribute to the public good, and many medical editors identify this aspect as a major satisfaction. Whether a medical editor's contribution helps a patient to address concerns, helps a researcher to share new findings and perhaps obtain a promotion, helps a clinician to provide effective care, helps a journalist to win an assignment or a prize, or helps a publisher to achieve high quality while containing costs, the work is valuable assistance.

The Five W's and an H of Medical Editing

Journalists often speak of presenting the five W's and an H: who, what, where, when, why, and how. These items also provide a good framework for considering the scope of medical editing.

WHO

For medical editing, *who* has multiple aspects. First, who enters medical editing? Medical editors come from a wide range of backgrounds. Many medical editors have degrees in English, journalism, or related areas. Many other medical editors have degrees in the sciences or health professions. Some of the best, and happiest, medical editors seem to be those who have long enjoyed both communication and science and find medical editing a fine way to combine their interests. For decades, people have debated whether better medical editors come from the humanities or the sciences. A look at the field makes clear, though, that many excellent editors come from each.

People also enter medical editing at a variety of career stages. Some do so shortly after earning an undergraduate degree. Others complete a master's degree in science journalism or a related field to prepare for such work. Still others obtain graduate degrees in the sciences or other realms and enter medical editing instead of a research-intensive or teaching-intensive career. Some physicians and other health professionals choose medical editing soon after receiving their degrees or after several years of clinical work. Some people move to medical editing in mid-career (for example, after working as a medical writer) or after retirement. Some people do medical editing part-time, either within a job that includes other duties or in addition to their main employment. People entering medical editing at different career stages can bring different assets—ranging from the latest academic knowledge, to laboratory or clinical experience, to transferable skills from working in corporate or other settings.

Much more important than your academic major or career stage is the ability to identify gaps in your knowledge and continually keep learning, both about editing and about medical subject matter. Other common features of successful medical editors include interest in medical content, enjoyment of language, attentiveness to detail, a problem-solving mentality, an ability to intuit what writers are trying to say, and a gift for intuiting how readers may interpret what was said. As in many fields, a sense of humor helps. In addition, an ability to work alone but also to interact well with others tends to mark the effective medical editor.

Something that tends *not* to mark the editor is a need for extensive credit. Granted, the contributions of medical editors should be openly recognized—for example, in the acknowledgments sections of scientific papers that they edit before journal submission and on the mastheads of journals for which they serve on the staff. However, medical editors tend to work mainly behind the scenes and to derive their satisfaction largely from helping others and from the improvement their work provides. It's the author who receives top billing.

Just as medical editors come from a wide range of disciplines, they also come from a variety of native languages. The assumption often is made that English-language medical editors must be native speakers of English. Many fine such editors, however, have other first languages. Also, much medical editing is in languages other than English. For English-language medical editing, the editor needs full English-language proficiency, which does not always equate to being a native speaker. And since medical editing often entails much more than correcting language, other aspects of the editor's abilities often are important.

Another part of *who*, bordering on the *what*, regards various categories of medical editors, or editorial roles. Major types of editors include the following:

- At a journal, the *editor-in-chief* provides overall leadership, especially regarding choice of content. Typically, the editor-in-chief of a biomedical journal is a prominent health professional or biomedical scientist and has published extensively as a researcher. Except at the largest and wealthiest journals, this position usually is part-time and pursued in conjunction with an academic or other appointment. Typically, medical journals also have *associate editors*, *assistant editors*, or such. Like the editor-in-chief, these editors tend to be active in research, to devote just part of their time to the journal, and to focus mainly on content. Together, these editors and the editor-in-chief are sometimes classified as *scientific editors*, given their emphasis on the scientific content rather than the writing. Magazines also have editors-in-chief, who likewise oversee the content of the publication as a whole.
- At entities that publish books, *acquisitions editors* obtain book proposals, guide authors in developing book manuscripts, and

oversee the decision whether to publish. Some book proposals or manuscripts arrive unsolicited. However, successful acquisitions editors also keep up with their subject areas (for example, by reading medical journals and attending medical conferences) and actively seek submissions from promising authors. Thus, biomedical background can be a considerable asset for a medical acquisitions editor.

- *Managing editors* manage the process of editing and publication. Thus, they may be concerned with items such as tracking, scheduling, staffing, and budgeting. Strong organizational skills therefore are needed. So are good interpersonal communication skills, as a managing editor may communicate extensively with authors and peer reviewers, as well as fellow members of the editorial team. However, subject-matter proficiency or language finesse may be less important than in some other editorial roles. In small editorial offices, a single individual may have both managing editor and manuscript editor duties, or a single individual may function as both managing editor and production editor.
- *Production editors* manage the transformation of a manuscript to a published product. Thus, depending on the type of publication, they may coordinate the work of manuscript editors, illustrators, designers, indexers, proofreaders, printers (and the electronic equivalent), and others. In addition, their job sometimes includes enlisting freelance contractors for such roles. Excellent organizational and interpersonal skills, as well as a broad knowledge of the editing and publishing processes, tend to be assets for production editors.
- *Manuscript editors*, also known as *copyeditors*, refine written materials. They may do so before or after the materials are submitted for publication or other dissemination. Perhaps most obviously, they ensure that mechanics such as grammar, spelling, punctuation, and word usage are correct; for medical copyediting, doing so can

Who's Who: Some Categories of Medical Editors

Acquisitions editor: editor in charge of acquiring and evaluating book manuscripts
Editor-in-chief: editor in charge of content of a journal, magazine, or other publication
Managing editor: editor in charge of administrative items such as scheduling, staffing, and budgeting
Manuscript editor: editor refining written materials for mechanics (such as grammar, spelling, and punctuation) and sometimes in other regards
Production editor: editor overseeing transformation of a manuscript to a published product

include checking use of medical terminology. If the writing is intended for publication, manuscript editors also may need to ensure that the writing complies with the publisher's requirements for style and format. For example, for many journals, they must edit manuscripts for consistency with American Medical Association style. Likewise, for other types of documents—such as grant proposals, presentation abstracts, and submissions to regulatory agencies—they may need to ensure that the writing meets the requirements of the recipient, such as the National Institutes of Health (which provides grants for biomedical research) or the Food and Drug Administration (which approves new drugs). Perhaps less obviously, manuscript editors' duties often extend to such matters as ensuring that writing is clear, complete, logical, concise, unbiased, and otherwise suitable. Manuscript editors may also help make sure that medical writing complies with ethical standards. As manuscript editors ultimately serve readers, they help suit the writing for the intended audience. In short, manuscript editors strive to ensure that writing communicates well.

The current book focuses mainly on providing guidance in medical manuscript editing. However, manuscript editors often interact with other categories of editors. Understanding their roles can help manuscript editors work effectively.

WHAT

Medical editors edit a wide variety of materials, ranging from technical reports to tweets. Most such editors focus mainly on one or another part of this spectrum.

Much medical editing is of technical materials for readers such as health professionals, biomedical researchers, and health policy specialists. Often such editing is of journal articles presenting new research. Another area of technical medical editing is regulatory editing: editing documents that companies submit to government agencies for approval of technologies such as drugs and medical devices. Other technical writings that medical editors may edit include grant proposals to obtain funding for biomedical research, textbooks and other learning materials for health-professional students and others, oral and poster presentations, and questions for the examinations used in licensing and certifying physicians and other health professionals.

Medical editing also can entail editing material for general audiences. Items that may be edited include medical articles for newspapers, magazines, and newsletters; medical books for the public; health-related web content from hospitals, clinics, health science centers, government agencies, health-related associations, and other sources; and posts for social media. Medical editors also may edit the scripts for videos, audio segments, or podcasts—or may edit such audiovisuals after production. They may also edit items such as informed-consent documents, patient-education materials, and resources intended to help keep healthy people from needing to become patients.

In addition, medical editing can include editing materials used in medical public relations, marketing, and advertising. The materials may be intended for the medical community, segments of the public, current or prospective investors or funders, or others. Examples include news releases, marketing brochures, and annual reports.

This book will deal most extensively with editing journal articles. However, it also will discuss editing other types of items. Much of the guidance on editing journal articles will apply to other medical editing as well.

WHEN

Medical editing can occur at various stages of a document's development. The nature of the editing varies accordingly. Early on, a medical editor may be involved in brainstorming about content and organization. Similarly, in editing an early draft, editing generally should address large-scale and medium-scale aspects rather than dwelling on copyeditorial details; it makes little sense to carefully polish text that might well be recast or deleted. Later, as a document approaches submission, publication, or posting, the editing rightly focuses on fine-scale aspects such as wording, mechanics, and the required style and format.

Some medical editors concentrate on editing materials at a given phase of development. Others edit materials at various phases. The distinction can depend in part on where a medical editor works—the subject of the next section.

WHERE

Medical editors work in a wide range of settings. These settings include publications and publishing companies. In particular, many medical editors work at journals. There, they may be editors-in-chief (or other editors in charge of content), managing editors, production editors, or manuscript editors. Some journals outsource manuscript editing to companies providing copyeditorial services; thus, some medical editors work for such companies. Medical editors also work for book publishers and companies providing editorial services for them. Some work for magazines or other popular media.

In addition, medical editors are employed at various institutions. These institutions include health-professional schools, health science centers, hospitals, clinics, health-related government agencies (such as the US National Institutes of Health, the US Centers for Disease Control and Prevention, and similar entities in other countries), international agencies such as the World Health Organization and the Pan American Health Organization, and other health-related organizations (such as the American Heart Association, the American Cancer Society, and many other disease-related associations worldwide). In such settings, medical editors commonly edit materials such as news releases, web content, and social media postings; they may also edit newsletters and magazines for their constituencies. Some serve as *author's editors*, helping researchers at their institutions to refine journal manuscripts or grant proposals before submission.

Medical editors also work in industry, most notably at pharmaceutical, biotechnology, and medical device companies. Here too they may assume a variety of roles. Some edit regulatory submissions and other documentation. Others edit materials intended to be read by journalists, health professionals, or the public. In addition, some medical editors work for public relations agencies or advertising agencies.

Many medical editors freelance, either instead of serving an employer or in addition to such work. Some freelance medical editors edit mainly specific types of medical writing, such as journal articles, grant proposals, or regulatory items. Others edit a variety of materials. Some do both freelance editing and freelance writing. Often, freelance medical editors have first obtained experience as editorial employees at journals, research institutions, or companies.

Geographically, the *where* for medical editors has been expanding. Traditionally, jobs for medical editors have tended to cluster largely in regions where many employers of medical editors are based—for example, the US Northeast, the Chicago area, and California. Increasingly, though, employers of medical editors have been offering remote opportunities. Thus, not only freelance but also other options can exist regardless of a medical editor's location.

WHY

The question "Why medical editing?" can be construed at least two ways. First, why pursue a career in medical editing? Second, why bother editing medical writing?

Medical editing has been called an accidental profession—for a common story is that of the liberal arts graduate who happens to obtain a job as a medical editor, turns out to like the work and excel in it, and pursues a career in the field. Other times, entry is less accidental. For example, many people who struggled to choose between a science career and a communication one are happy to find that medical editing is both. Other appeals of medical editing, for both accidental and not-so-accidental medical editors, include the chance to continually learn. The diversity of working arrangements available also attracts and helps retain some medical editors—for options range from part-time through full-time-plus, from largely individual through largely team-based, and from solely remote through solely onsite. And as noted, the chance to contribute to medicine and health can be a major appeal.

As for why bother editing medical writing: Manuscript editors often express the rationale for their work in terms of multiple C's. These tend to include clarity, correctness, consistency, completeness, conciseness, and courtesy. For medical editors, all are important.

- *Clarity* is paramount. Ultimately, the editor's role is to help ensure effective communication. Thus, when faced with a choice between clarity and another C (such as conciseness), the editor should choose clarity. To edit for clarity, an editor must be able to discern (or ask) what the author is trying to say. And an editor must be able to sense how readers will interpret what was said. Editing for clarity is especially important in editing medical materials, as misinterpretation could cause literal harm.
- Editing for *correctness* in various regards also is fundamental. Of course, such editing includes correcting errors in grammar, spelling, punctuation, word usage, and other mechanics. It also extends further. Although editors of medical text usually are not expected to be experts on the content, they should (tactfully) ask authors

about items that appear likely to be incorrect—for example, numbers that seem implausible. They also should query if the reasoning in a passage seems incorrect or obscure.

- Medical editors also edit for *consistency*. Among other things: The information should be consistent throughout (rather than, for instance, differing between tables and text). Conclusions should be consistent with evidence presented. Formatting should be consistent throughout. The piece should comply with conventions in the field (such as those regarding medical nomenclature) and with conventions regarding content and structure of given types of documents. And the writing should comply with the instructions provided by, for example, the journal or granting agency. Medical editors check for consistency in all such regards.
- *Completeness* is another aspect to address. Does anything seem to be missing? At the other extreme, is anything present that doesn't seem to belong? In either case, the editor should flag the matter and consult the author.
- *Conciseness* (or concision)—in other words, brevity—is important for multiple reasons. First, writing that is concise tends to be clearer, and it is faster to read—a major consideration for busy medical readers. Because shorter writing looks less intimidating, it is more likely to indeed be read. Also, concise wording helps medical writing convey the needed information while still complying with constraints such as word limits for journal articles or page limits for proposals. Accordingly, a common task of a medical editor is to make writing more concise.
- Not all lists of editorial C's include *courtesy*. In medical editing, though, courtesy in various regards deserves attention. For example, medical editors should help ensure that wording is respectful to people with diseases or disabilities and that, more generally, language is inclusive and otherwise unbiased. They should, of course, be courteous and respectful in their interactions with authors. And they should strive to ensure that the writing respects the intelligence, time, and priorities of readers.

HOW

How can medical writers attain the multiple C's? How can they find professional opportunities that suit them? How can they continue to develop professionally and keep obtaining satisfaction from their work? Addressing such questions will be the main focus of the rest of this book.

A Partnership with Authors, Readers, and More

As shown in this chapter, medical editing is a profession of broad scope in various regards. Medical editors occupy a wide range of niches. In many contexts, they must recognize authors' motivations for writing, grasp what authors are trying to say, and help them say it in ways that are comfortable to them and that suit publishers and readers. Commonly, they must understand and work with stylistic, financial, and other concerns of publishers or other entities. Perhaps most important, they must sense how readers will interpret what is said, understand how readers can best grasp the content, and serve as advocates for readers' right to sound and accessible information. Accordingly, medical editors are partners with various constituencies.

Thus, contrary to the stereotype, medical editors are much more than unsociable, inflexible wretches grimly correcting grammar in journal articles. Although many are fairly quiet and most are comfortable working largely alone, good medical editors are sensitive to the feelings and needs of others and can communicate accordingly and help others do so. Although well versed in grammatical and other relevant norms, they have the flexibility to override such norms when compliance would interfere with effective communication. They may edit any of a wide range of materials for any of a wide range of audiences. Commonly, they derive fulfillment from their craft and their careers.

Finally, medical editing is a welcoming profession. Demand for skilled medical editors exceeds supply, and medical editors generally welcome new colleagues, mentor their less experienced counterparts, and help each other rather than compete. If you already do medical editing, I hope this characterization concurs with your experience. And if you have not yet entered the medical editing community, please let me welcome you.

Key Points

- Medical editing is a helping profession, serving readers, authors, and publishers.
- Medical editors come from a wide variety of backgrounds, including communication fields, the sciences, and the health professions.

- Medical editors may edit a wide variety of materials. Examples include journal articles, grant proposals, regulatory documents, and items for general readers.
- Medical editors work in varied settings. Among them are journals, academic institutions, government agencies, and health-related corporations. Some medical editors freelance.
- Rationales for medical editing include clarity, correctness, consistency, completeness, conciseness, and courtesy.

· 2 ·

Key Resources for Medical Editors

Medical editors—and medical-editors-to-be—have many resources to draw on. These sometimes interrelated resources include medical style manuals and other key books, professional organizations and their publications, educational programs, online resources, and medical editing colleagues. This chapter provides an overview of some major such resources. Such resources can help fledgling medical editors develop knowledge and skills in the profession. They also can help established medical editors keep up with evolving style norms, advancing medical knowledge, emerging editorial technologies, new career opportunities, and more. In addition, medical editors continually consult such resources for guidance in their work. Thus, medical editors employ such resources throughout their careers. Obtaining access to such resources and becoming familiar with what they offer constitute a fine investment.

Style Manuals in Medicine and Related Realms

A medical editor's literal or figurative bookshelf should include a style manual—or, more likely, several. Especially if you will edit journal articles or other scholarly or technical medical writings, the *AMA [American Medical Association] Manual of Style* (AMA Manual of Style Committee 2020) generally merits a central position. Other style manuals that often deserve a place include *The CSE [Council of Science Editors] Manual:*

Scientific Style and Format for Authors, Editors, and Publishers (Council of Science Editors Style Manual Task Force 2024), the *Publication Manual of the American Psychological Association* (American Psychological Association 2020), and *The Chicago Manual of Style* (University of Chicago Press Editorial Staff 2024). For editing news articles, news releases, and some other materials for general readerships, *The Associated Press Stylebook* (Associated Press 2024) is standard. Other style manuals that medical editors may find useful include the US Government Printing Office style manual (US Government Printing Office 2016) and the *ACS [American Chemical Society] Guide to Scholarly Communication* (Banik et al. 2020).

Style manuals also are called style guides. As stated by the Purdue Online Writing Lab, style guides "include a wide range of rules and guidelines for works in their respective fields" (Purdue Online Writing Lab, n.d.). On the mechanical level, they address questions such as the following: Which conventions should you follow for punctuation? (For example, should you write "measles, mumps and chicken pox" or "measles, mumps, and chicken pox"—with the serial comma included?) What rules should you follow regarding when to write numbers as words and when to present them as numerals? What formats should you use to cite references in text and to present them in a reference list? In addition, style manuals in medicine and science often contain guidance specific to the discipline. Examples include information on standard nomenclature (terminology) in specific areas of research or clinical care, lists of accepted biomedical abbreviations, and material on publication ethics in medicine and science.

In addition, some style manuals, such as *The Chicago Manual of Style* and *The CSE Manual*, contain guidance on indexing. This guidance can aid in editing indexes. Some medical editors turn out to have such a proclivity for indexing that they end up doing some indexing themselves.

Major style manuals in medicine, the sciences, and other fields generally are available both in print and online. Many medical editors like to have access to both, either as personal copies or through libraries. Online copies usually are easy to search, tend to be continually updated, and sometimes contain supplemental material unavailable in print. Personal print copies are easy to bookmark physically and to annotate; frequently consulted sections can be readily accessed. Websites associated with style manuals commonly list updates made since the current print version appeared. If you are using a print version, check periodically for such updates. Of course, regardless of whether you are using a style manual online or in print, be sure to use the current edition.

THE AMA MANUAL OF STYLE

Currently in its 11th edition, the *AMA Manual of Style: A Guide for Authors and Editors* is the predominant style manual for editing medical journal articles in the United States. Many US journals in human medicine, veterinary medicine, and related fields follow AMA style, either entirely or with journal-specific adaptations. Some aspects of this manual's content—such as the material on ethical considerations and on study design and statistics—also can aid editors of manuscripts for medical journals in languages other than English or following other styles. Likewise, much of the content can provide guidance in editing medical writing other than journal articles.

Running some 1200 pages in print (including the index), the *AMA Manual* contains chapters both on style per se and on other aspects of medical writing, editing, and publishing. Among the chapters that medical manuscript editors might find useful to consult most often are those on grammar, punctuation, capitalization, word usage, abbreviations, nomenclature, numbers and percentages, tables and figures, and references. The chapters on topics such as grammar and punctuation contain medical examples to illustrate the points.

Consulting the *AMA Manual* can resolve many questions that arise in editing medical manuscripts. Some examples: Should *case* or *patient* be used in a given instance? Should a manuscript say *Alzheimer's disease* or *Alzheimer disease*? Was an author correct to use numerals even for numbers less than 10? Did an author designate blood groups, cancer stages, or heart murmurs in the proper way? Are all the references in the reference list formatted appropriately?

Other parts of the *AMA Manual* that medical manuscript editors may do well to consult include the chapters on manuscript preparation, units of measure, and study design and statistics. Ditto for the glossary of publishing terms and the resource list. The manual also contains a lengthy chapter (more than 200 pages!) on ethical and legal considerations, ranging from responsibilities of authors and editors, to scientific misconduct, to intellectual property topics such as copyright. This chapter can provide valuable browsing for new and not-so-new medical editors, and the chapter on types of articles (such as research reports, review articles, and opinion pieces) may help introduce newcomers to editing manuscripts for medical journals. Because a style manual is a reference work, it is not meant to be read from cover to cover. However, reading or skimming sections from time to time can alert editors to issues for which to be on the lookout, increase editors' awareness of what the manual can help with, and contribute more generally to initial or continuing editorial education.

For editorial education, the online version of the *AMA Manual* includes quizzes on many topics the manual covers. The forerunners of the current quizzes originated years ago, when experienced manuscript editors at the American Medical Association developed quizzes to help train new manuscript editors at journals published by the association. I learned of these quizzes at a conference and requested copies, which I received on the condition that they be used only in teaching my students. Eventually, as the broader value of the quizzes became clear and as the online version of the *AMA Manual* emerged, these quizzes became available through the journal website. Over the years, the quizzes have been updated, and new quizzes have been added. Although the website still terms the quizzes "style quizzes," current topics of the quizzes include not only style in the narrow sense (for example, capitalization, grammar, plurals, and references) but also topics such as ethics, figure and table design, inclusive language, intellectual property, and editing material within specific medical fields (such as cardiology, neurology, and ophthalmology). These quizzes tend to be extensive and to have answer keys with detailed explanations. Taking the quizzes and reviewing the answer keys can constitute essentially a course in medical copyediting.

New editions of the *AMA Manual* have tended to emerge about once a decade. However, the manual is continually updated, in keeping with changes in medicine, language, scientific communication, and society. Updates appear in the update section of the manual's website (https://academic.oup.com/amamanualofstyle/pages/about/updates-to-the-manual). Examples of updates since early 2020, when the 11th edition of the manual was released, include recommendations for reporting use of artificial intelligence (AI); entries on COVID-19 terminology; updates on hyphenation, on citation of preprints, and on reporting race and ethnicity; addition of a policy on authors' requests to have their names changed on papers after publication; and additional guidance on citing items presented at virtual or hybrid meetings. The medical editor's world keeps evolving, and the manual keeps evolving accordingly.

SOME OTHER STYLE MANUALS USEFUL TO MEDICAL EDITORS

Medical editors can benefit from access to multiple style manuals. One reason is that not all journals that publish medical research (and not all other venues presenting medical content) follow the same style. Although AMA style dominates, its use is not imperative, and some publications find that other conventions better suit their content, media, readerships, or traditions. Another reason is that no one style manual can be truly comprehensive; thus, even when a medical editor uses primarily a given style manual for a given endeavor, occasion can arise to consult others.

The CSE Manual, from the Council of Science Editors, can especially aid in editing materials in the basic medical sciences, as it includes chapters on special conventions followed in respective fields of science. Among chapters that may be especially relevant in this regard are those on drugs and pharmacokinetics and on genes, chromosomes, and related molecules. In addition, the book contains a chapter on disease names. Regarding mechanics, such as whether to use the serial comma and when to present numbers as numerals, CSE style tends to resemble AMA style. Thus, switching between the styles usually is relatively easy.

In the social and behavioral sciences, journals commonly follow APA (American Psychological Association) style. Thus, editing materials on social and behavioral aspects of medicine and health sometimes entails using this style. The *Publication Manual of the American Psychological Association* and its companion website (at https://apastyle.apa.org), which includes supplemental content, are the authoritative resources on this style. Unlike the *AMA Manual* and *The CSE Manual*, this manual is not available online. However, the manual is available as an ebook, as well as in print. The print edition is available in a version that, conveniently, is spiral bound and has thumb tabs.

For book publishing in the United States, and more generally as a handbook of scholarly editing, *The Chicago Manual of Style* merits its cover line as "the essential guide for writers, editors, and publishers." Editors of books on medical topics often employ Chicago style or an adaptation thereof. And editors following other styles often find it helpful to consult the Chicago manual about specialized aspects of writing style that style manuals in medicine or science do not address as thoroughly or at all. The book also includes helpful guidance on the manuscript editing process.

Medical editors also may find it useful to consult the *ACS Guide to Scholarly Communication*, a continually updated online-only manual from the American Chemical Society. Some parts of this manual, such as those on chemical structures and chemical nomenclature, can aid in editing materials on chemically related medical topics. Other parts of the manual can aid more generally in editing scientific content and guiding authors.

US newspapers typically follow AP (Associated Press) style, on which the *AP Stylebook* provides detailed guidance. Many other materials for general readers also follow this style or a variant of it. Thus, editors of lay materials on medical topics commonly consult this style manual, which is available in print and as a continually updated online edition. In particular, editors of news stories or news releases often must ensure that the work is in proper AP style. Of special relevance in medical editing: The *AP Stylebook* now includes a section on covering health and science, and its guidance on writing about disabilities has expanded greatly. Perhaps the most apparent difference of AP style from AMA, CSE, APA, and Chicago style is as follows: In most contexts, AP style does not employ the serial comma.

Some publications or institutions have their own style manuals—or their own supplements to standard style manuals. Such supplements may specify deviations from the main style manual used (for example, different preferences regarding the spelling of certain terms). They may also present items such as terminology specific to the topic area of the journal or to aspects of the institution. When editing for a given periodical or institution, such supplements can be worth checking for.

Other Books

What else might a medical editor's bookshelf contain? The answer can depend in part on the background of the editor, the type of editing done, and the editor's tastes. However, a medical editor should have access to a medical dictionary. Over the years, two giants in the field—both literally and figuratively—have been *Dorland's Illustrated Medical Dictionary* and *Stedman's Medical Dictionary*. Traditionally, these two books have been massive tomes. Now, however, they are principally online products available by subscription. (See https://www.dorlandsonline.com/dorland/home and https://www.wolterskluwer.com/en/solutions/lippincott-medicine/medical-education/stedmans-online-medical-dictionary.) These dictionaries contain some entries so extensive that they resemble encyclopedia articles. Multiple other medical dictionaries also exist. They include both general medical dictionaries and dictionaries in specific health professions (such as dentistry, nursing, or veterinary medicine) and in various languages. There also are multilingual medical dictionaries and specialized works such as dictionaries of medical acronyms and abbreviations. Spell-checkers associated with medical dictionaries can be of considerable help.

Of course, medical editors also need access to general dictionaries. For consistency, medical journals and other entities commonly specify the dictionary that editors working for them should use. One commonly recommended dictionary is *Merriam-Webster's Collegiate Dictionary*, which is continually updated and can be accessed at https://www.merriam-webster.com/. In addition, many editors bookmark the website One-Look Dictionary Search (https://onelook.com/), which enables searching of multiple dictionaries at once.

For individuals entering medical editing from backgrounds other than the health professions, medical terminology books—especially those designed for self-study—can aid in establishing a firm foundation. Such a book, *Elements of Medical Terminology* (Gastel 2010), is available as part of the American Medical Writers Association's "essential skills" workbook series (https://www.amwa.org/page/ES_Certificate). Within this series, the workbooks on grammar and usage, punctuation, and sentence structure may especially suit beginning medical editors who come from science backgrounds and lack formal training in English. The remaining three books in the series—on ethics, statistics, and tables and graphs—can serve medical editors from a variety of backgrounds.

Excellent briefings on punctuation, grammar, and related subjects appear in *The Copyeditor's Handbook* (Einsohn and Schwartz 2019). This comprehensive guide also addresses many other aspects of mechanics, such as spelling, hyphenation, capitalization, and abbreviations. In addition, it provides comprehensive, authoritative guidance on tasks and procedures in copyediting. And it identifies many helpful reference books and other resources. Although a few parts of this book, such as that on quotations, may not be very relevant to most medical editors, overall the book is key reading for beginning medical (or other) copyeditors. Even experienced editors are likely to gain new knowledge and insights from this book and to find it useful to consult.

An accompanying resource, *The Copyeditor's Workbook* (Bűky, Schwartz, and Einsohn 2019), contains exercises for the various chapters of *The Copyeditor's Handbook*. Like the quizzes accompanying the *AMA Manual of Style*, these exercises have detailed keys containing extensive explanation. Although few of the exercises in *The Copyeditor's Workbook* have medically related content, almost all of the exercises help cultivate skills useful in medical editing.

For a broader, more philosophical perspective on copyediting, *The Subversive Copy Editor: Advice from Chicago (or, How to Negotiate Good Relationships with Your Writers, Your Colleagues, and Yourself)* (Saller 2016), by Carol Fisher Saller of the University of Chicago Press, has much to offer. Written with wisdom and wit, this book addresses topics ranging from how to work effectively and amicably with authors, to how to prioritize tasks and issues, to how to cope with editorial errors or lapses (which inevitably occur, as no editor is perfect). Although the book ends with a chapter on breaking into the copyediting field, it can resonate with editors at various career stages. Indeed, like many good writings, this book can have different significance to readers at different stages of professional or personal maturity.

Medical textbooks can be useful to consult, for example when editing manuscripts on unfamiliar medical topics. For clinical medicine, standard general medical texts include the Merck Manuals (https://www.merckmanuals.com/), of which professional, consumer, and veterinary versions exist. Conveniently, the Merck Manuals are fully accessible online at no cost and are available in English, Spanish, and several other languages. Editors who regularly edit manuscripts in particular medical specialties or subspecialties—such as cardiology, gastroenterology, or neurosurgery—may find it useful to have textbooks in those areas. Likewise, editors focusing on specific fields of basic medical science—such as microbiology, neuroscience, or pharmacology—can benefit from having textbooks in those fields to consult.

Books on medical writing, or more generally scientific writing, can help round out the medical editor's bookshelf. Such books can serve two major functions. First, they can acquaint the medical editor with norms and expectations such as those for the structure of journal articles reporting medical research. Second, they can be helpful to suggest to authors or to cite as authorities when suggesting revisions. Many good such books exist. Four by authors who are experienced in medical editing, and thus whose books may reflect particular awareness in this realm, are *Essentials of Writing Biomedical Research Papers*, by Mimi Zeiger (2000); *How to Write, Publish, and Present in the Health Sciences: A Guide for Clinicians and Laboratory Researchers*, by Thomas A. Lang (2010); *How to Write and Publish a Scientific Paper*, by Barbara Gastel and Robert A. Day (2022); and *Avoiding Common Pitfalls in Medical Writing: An Editor's Advice*, by Deanna Erin Conners (2024). Also of note is *Principles of Scientific Writing and Biomedical Publication: A JAMA Editors' Guide for Authors* (Fontanarosa, Flanagin, and Greenland 2024). Although its most recent edition appeared in the year 2000, the Zeiger book remains a fine resource, especially for editing papers in the basic medical sciences. Of particular value, this book contains exercises, most of which entail editing. The Lang book, which is more general, discusses not only writing journal articles but also preparing grant proposals, poster presentations, and slides. Another book from Lang, *How to Report Statistics in Medicine: Annotated Guidelines for Authors, Editors, and Reviewers* (Lang and Secic 2006), also is a valuable reference. The book by Gastel and Day, which includes chapters on the parts of a scientific paper, has grown in scope to address other types of writing as well. The Conners book, which is openly accessible at https://milneopentextbooks.org/avoiding-ariou-pitfalls-in-medical-writing/, consists of fact sheets on various aspects of academic medical writing, publishing, and presenting, including recent topics such as search engine optimization. The fact sheets can be useful to consult and to share with authors. The *JAMA* guide includes chapters by many experienced journal editors. Medical writing books largely for medical practitioners—for example, *Medical Writing: A Guide for Clinicians, Educators, and Researchers* (Taylor 2018)—can aid especially in editing materials specific to clinical medicine, such as case reports. Also, for those editing regulatory medical writing, *Regulatory Writing: An Overview* (DeTora 2020), from the Regulatory Affairs Professionals Society, can be a useful resource.

Finally, medical editors who freelance can benefit from books providing guidance to freelancers and, more generally, owners of small businesses. *The Chicago Guide for Freelance Editors* (Brenner 2024) addresses many aspects of the topic, such as deciding to freelance, setting rates, branding oneself, marketing, setting up a workspace, handling files, keeping records, and managing difficult situations. Another book to consider is *What to Charge: Pricing Strategies for Freelancers and Consultants*, by medical writer and editor Laurie Lewis (Lewis 2011). Other sources of guidance for freelancers and others include resources from, and contacts through, professional associations—the topic of the next section.

Professional Organizations and Their Publications

Medical editors tend to be a congenial community, eager to welcome and help each other. However, this community is highly dispersed. Although some medical editors work with multiple peers at journals or elsewhere, many are the only medical editors at their institutions or in their departments, and many do solely freelance work. Even in units with multiple medical editors, remote work has become common. So, how do medical editors establish and maintain their community? Largely through professional organizations and the relationships developed through them. In addition, these organizations provide medical writers with instruction, help them keep up with the field, alert them to employment opportunities, and more.

Commonly, medical editors belong to organizations more broadly for science editors or medical communicators. These organizations offer many resources. They generally have highly informative *websites*, with substantial parts open to nonmembers. They have *periodicals* and other publications. They have *conferences*—in person, online, or hybrid—at which attendees can increase their knowledge and network with colleagues. They have *webinars* and other online events. They post *job announcements*. They have *email discussion lists* and *online forums* through which members can ask questions, note resources, and otherwise communicate. Some also have other offerings, such as courses and certificates.

In North America, the Council of Science Editors (CSE; https://www.councilscienceeditors.org/) is the predominant organization for medical and other scientific editors. Known until the year 2000 as the Council of Biology Editors, CSE has medical editors as a very sizeable component. Resources from CSE include *The CSE Manual: Scientific Style and Format for Authors, Editors, and Publishers* (2024); the periodical *Science Editor*; the continually updated *Recommendations for Promoting Integrity in Scientific Journal Publications* (Council of Science Editors Editorial Policy Committee, n.d.); short courses on manuscript editing and other topics; and a mentorship program, as well as an annual conference, webinars, and other events. Distinctively, CSE's online postings of job opportunities are accessible even to nonmembers.

CSE's counterpart based in Europe is the European Association of Science Editors (EASE; https://ease.org.uk/). Resources from EASE include its journal, *European Science Editing*; the EASE Science Editors' Handbook; the EASE Guidelines for Authors and Translators of Scientific Articles to be Published in English (freely available in 30 languages); and conferences and other events. Both CSE and EASE include members from outside the continents on which they are based. Indeed, EASE has regional chapters both within and outside Europe.

Organizations of science editors, including medical editors, also exist in other countries and regions. Examples include the Asian Council of Science Editors (https://theacse.com/), Associação Brasileira de Editores Científicos (the Brazilian Association of Scientific Editors; https://www.abecbrasil.org.br/novo/), the Council of Asian Science Editors (https://www.asianeditor.org/), and the Korean Council of Science Editors (https://kcse.org/).

Some organizations of medically related editors serve largely editors determining journal content, rather than manuscript editors or others. Prominent among them is the World Association of Medical Editors (WAME, pronounced "whammy"; https://www.wame.org/index.php). Although only decision-making editors at peer-reviewed medical journals and selected medical editing scholars can join this free organization, anyone interested can access much of its website. Other groups largely for editors associated with journals include the American Association of Dental Editors and Journalists (AADEJ; https://www.aadej.org/) and the International Academy of Nursing Editors (or—yes, that's true—INANE; https://nursingeditors.com/).

Consisting primarily of members editing grant proposals or scientific papers in the

---

Some Organizations for Medical Editors to Consider

ORGANIZATIONS IN SCIENCE EDITING:

- Council of Science Editors
- European Association of Science Editors
- Scientific Editors Network

OTHER ORGANIZATIONS TO CONSIDER:

- ACES: The Society for Editing
- American Medical Writers Association
- Association of Health Care Journalists
- Drug Information Association
- Editorial Freelancers Association
- International Society for Medical Publication Professionals
- National Association of Science Writers
- Regulatory Affairs Professionals Society

United States, the Scientific Editors Network, or ScENe (https://www.scientificeditorsnetwork.org/), began as an informal group expanding through personal contacts. However, the network now accepts applications for membership. The network's core activity remains monthly online meetings focusing on topics in scientific, including medical, editing. The network also has an active email discussion list.

Despite the "writers" in its name, the American Medical Writers Association (AMWA; https://www.amwa.org/) is a broad-based organization for medical communication professionals, and it includes many medical editors. Its resources include the *AMWA Journal* (which often has editorially related content), the Essential Skills modules (the set of which can be completed to earn a certificate), an annual conference, and many online educational events. In addition, AMWA has regional chapters, and it offers a certification examination. Whereas CSE and EASE focus largely on editing journal articles and journals, AMWA ranges more widely and has many members involved in regulatory writing and editing. Much on medical communication careers is available in the AMWA "Ultimate Guide to Becoming a Medical Writer" (https://info.amwa.org/ultimate-guide-to-becoming-a-medical-writer), posted on the AMWA website.

The Board of Editors in the Life Sciences (BELS; https://www.bels.org/) mainly administers an examination to certify individuals as proficient in life science editing, which includes medical editing. Its website includes a directory of individuals who have thus been certified. Over the years since its founding in 1991, BELS also has evolved into a professional organization for editors with BELS certification. Thus, for example, it has a newsletter, an email discussion list, and online events. It also has occasional gatherings in conjunction with conferences such as those of AMWA or CSE.

Some medical editors join—or at least consult websites of—organizations in related fields or general editing organizations. Well-established general editing organizations include ACES: The Society for Editing (https://aceseditors.org/) and the Editorial Freelancers Association (EFA; https://www.the-efa.org/). For editors of medical writing for general readerships, organizations such as the Association of Health Care Journalists (AHCJ; https://healthjournalism.org/) and the National Association of Science Writers (NASW; https://www.nasw.org/) can be helpful. And editors of medical regulatory materials can benefit from groups such as the Drug Information Association (DIA; https://www.diaglobal.org/), the International Society for Medical Publication Professionals (ISMPP; https://www.ismpp.org/), and the Regulatory Affairs Professionals Society (RAPS; https://www.raps.org/).

How can fledgling medical editors make best use of the organizations available? Browsing through some of the organizations' websites can be an excellent start. Without investing anything other than time, you can thereby learn much about the field and see which organizations best suit your professional interests and personal style. Then join one of the organizations, or maybe two or three; if you are still in school, you may qualify for a student membership rate. Rather than continuing to lurk, get involved. Attend, and network at, some face-to-face or virtual events. Volunteer for committees, which often want to involve new members. Offer to write for, or to otherwise help with, the association's publications. Ask and answer questions in associations' email discussion lists or other forums. In short, become an active part of the congenial community of medical editors. You are likely to learn much, form valuable ties, avoid professional isolation, and otherwise enrich your career.

Educational Opportunities

As noted, medical editors enter the field through widely varied paths. Few have had formal training in medical editing per se. Although the field tends to attract people with combined interests in medicine and communication, those from the liberal arts often have little medical background, and those from the sciences or health professions often have limited editorial knowledge. Thus, medical editors generally have learned their craft mainly on the job. Some have had expert medical editors as mentors. Others have relied largely on intelligence, instinct, and lots of looking things up to fill the gaps.

Fortunately, many resources now exist for initial and continuing education of medical editors. As noted, organizations in science editing and related fields offer self-study materials, workshops, short courses, webinars, mentorships, and more. In addition, relevant knowledge and skills can be gained through undergraduate and graduate courses and programs, extracurricular activities, non-degree certificate programs, and open online courses. Internships also can provide valuable experience and an entrée to the field.

If you are an undergraduate, graduate, or professional student thinking of a medical editing career, consider taking one or more courses that will round out your preparation. For instance, if you come from the liberal arts, perhaps take a medical terminology course and some health and science courses. If you are a science major, make room for an editing course, if available, and writing-intensive courses. If you have elective time as a health-professional student, consider arranging an experience in medical editing or a related realm; some faculty members in the medical humanities offer such experiences, and some medical journals have hosted medical students for rotations. Whatever your major, try to gain extracurricular experience on student publications. If your institution has a student science journal, working on it may be ideal. Ditto for involvement with publications such as *The Journal of Young Investigators* (https://www.jyi.org/). (Speaking of young investigators: Try to get some research experience while a student; doing so can increase both your insight and your empathy in editing reports of research.) Working on a student newspaper, yearbook, literary magazine, or medical humanities periodical also can foster relevant skills.

Many colleges and universities offer courses in *science writing* (in other words, writing for the public about science), *scientific writing* (scientist-to-scientist writing, such as journal articles and grant proposals), and related subjects. Some offer undergraduate or graduate majors in communicating science or in related fields, such as professional writing or technical writing. Such courses and majors can prepare students for medical editing careers. Links to information on some of the well-established programs appear in the AMWA guide to becoming a medical writer (at https://info.amwa.org/ultimate-guide-to-becoming-a-medical-writer#medical_writer_resources) and at https://ksj.mit.edu/resource/being-a-science-journalist/schools/ within the website of the Knight Science Journalism Program at MIT.

If you have already completed your formal education, you may still be able to take college or university courses to complement your background. Some universities allow college graduates to take courses as non-degree-seeking students. Also, consider taking courses at a community college. Such courses tend to be less expensive than those elsewhere, and often they are scheduled to suit registrants employed full-time.

For individuals already holding degrees, specialized certificate programs also can work well. Two that can especially suit aspiring or current medical editors are the University of Chicago certificate program in medical writing and editing (https://professional.uchicago.edu/find-your-fit/certificates/medical-writing-and-editing) and the University of California, San Diego, certificate program in medical writing (https://extendedstudies.ucsd.edu/courses-and-programs/medical-communication-courses). In these two programs, participants complete a series of online courses. The participants in such programs range from recent degree recipients, to mid-career professionals wanting to change their focus or enhance their abilities and credentials, to individuals hoping to edit or write after retiring from their primary careers.

Alternatively, people interested in medical editing have some freestanding online courses available. One is the medical editing course hosted by the Chartered Institute of Editing and Proofreading (see https://www.ciep.uk/learn-and-develop/training-courses/medical-editing-e-learning.html). Another is the Editorial Freelancers Association course "Introduction to Medical Editing and AMA Style" (https://www.the-efa.org/product/introduction-to-medical-editing-and-ama-style/).

Massive open online courses (MOOCs) can be a convenient—and free or inexpensive—way to round out knowledge in scientific communication, medical science, and other areas relevant to medical editing. For example, Coursera (https://www.coursera.org/), which includes noncredit online courses from multiple prominent universities, has courses in grammar and punctuation, biostatistics, clinical research, epidemiology, medical terminology, writing in the sciences, and a wide variety of other subjects. Also, Rising Scholars (https://risingscholars.net/en/), a program primarily for researchers in the Global South that was formerly known as AuthorAID, offers MOOCs on writing journal articles and grant proposals. In addition, the Rising Scholars online resource library includes materials that can help in medical editing and related work.

Finally, internships—where trainees receive practical experience in professional contexts—can facilitate the transition to a medical editing career. Among their benefits: Internships provide real-world opportunities to gain knowledge and develop skills. They are low-risk ways to see whether you like given types of work and given employers. Likewise, they allow employers to evaluate potential hires without making long-term commitments. They are a way to build credentials and generate work samples. Internship supervisors can serve as references and help in finding employment. Internships also can yield other contacts. And sometimes internships evolve into jobs. In short, internships can be a fine way to break in.

Internships in medical editing and related realms can be parts of formally established internship programs or experiences arranged ad hoc. Examples of settings where students have done internships in medical editing, medical writing, or a mix include the MD Anderson Cancer Center editorial office, US National Institutes of Health, US Centers for Disease Control and Prevention, pharmaceutical and biotechnology companies, universities, and companies providing editing services to authors. Some internships and fellowships are specifically for physicians wanting to explore medical editing and publishing. Full-time, yearlong editorial fellowships for physicians are available at the medical journal *JAMA* (https://jamanetwork.com/pages/fishbein-fellowship) and the *New England Journal of Medicine* (https://www.youtube.com/playlist?list=PLI8Ak-hj5dgFT5Y2yeoq5BU4EB28EL1H3). Journals or publishers with shorter-term or less intensive editorial fellowships for physicians and sometimes for PhDs have included the journal *American Family Physician*, the *Journal of General Internal Medicine*, the Radiological Society of North America, and the American Society of Clinical Oncology. Additional information appears in an article and associated table by medical editor Madison Semro (2023a, 2023b).

Whereas some editorial internships and fellowships are for specific groups—such as students or physicians—others are flexible in this regard. And whereas some are entirely on-site, some are now at least in part remote. Explore existing opportunities and their requirements, but do not feel limited by them. If an opportunity interests you, inquire; there may be some flexibility, or a related opportunity may be available. Likewise, if there's a setting where you think you would like to do an internship, inquire even if an internship has not been announced. Having seen your initiative, a medical editor might well be willing to accept you as an intern.

Online Resources

Online access to resources already mentioned, such as style manuals and medical dictionaries, can aid the medical editor. In addition, consider bookmarking other online resources that can merit frequent consultation. Given the fluidity of the online world, sometimes the URLs of such resources change or the resources become unavailable. In general, the online resources listed in this section and elsewhere in this book are well established and have long had stable URLs. If, however, a resource is not at the listed URL and you are not directed elsewhere, searching may be in order.

One resource popular among medical and other editors is OneLook

Dictionary Search (https://onelook.com/), which lets you look up words in multiple general and specialized dictionaries at once. As well as being a quick way to check spellings and definitions, OneLook can help when an individual dictionary does not include a particular use of a given word, or when it might be unclear from a single dictionary whether a word has been used correctly. Some dictionaries in OneLook not only write pronunciations phonetically but also include audio recordings of words—which can help in preparing to discuss manuscripts with authors.

Two resources from the US National Library of Medicine—PubMed and MedlinePlus—can be highly beneficial to bookmark. PubMed (https://pubmed.ncbi.nlm.nih.gov/), which covers most major English-language medical journals plus many other journals, is the predominant resource for searching the medical literature. To identify relevant journal articles, you can search PubMed using subject-matter terms, author names, and journal names; you can also narrow the search in various regards, such as by type of article (for example, review article or clinical trial) and by range of publication dates. PubMed searches yield bibliographic information, abstracts, and sometimes full text.

Medical editors can find PubMed searching helpful for various purposes. Most importantly, it can aid in gaining background on a topic before editing a manuscript. (Tip: Look for review articles on the topic.) It can reveal the publication history of authors whose work you will edit. (Knowing whether a manuscript is from a newbie or an experienced author can help guide interactions.) It can help show whether a term seems to be used correctly. (Advice: Look for articles on the same topic in well-edited major medical journals, such as *JAMA* and the *New England Journal of Medicine*.) Of course, it can help in following up when a reference seems likely to contain an error (for example, because a publication date seems unlikely).

MedlinePlus (https://medlineplus.gov/) provides health information mainly for the general public but can assist medical editors too. Among other things, it includes a medical encyclopedia, a section on medical tests, and a section on drugs and supplements. Perhaps most notably, searching it by subject yields carefully vetted lay materials from a variety of sources. Full-text and easy to understand, the materials can be helpful to consult before starting to edit a piece on an unfamiliar medical topic—or when seeking a refresher or update before looking at sources that are more technical. MedlinePlus also can help in editing materials for general readers by showing how the subject has been presented elsewhere. (By the way, editors wishing to sustain their body and spirit might also like the "healthy recipes" part of this website.)

Other US government resources include plainlanguage.gov (https://www.plainlanguage.gov/). This website, which includes guidelines and examples, can be especially helpful in editing materials to be readily understandable by general readerships. The principles also apply to helping to make writing readable for other audiences.

When editing a manuscript to submit to a specific journal, the editor should consult the journal's *instructions to authors*. These instructions should appear on the journal's website; if they do not, beware of the quality of the journal. Sometimes, however, the instructions are hard to locate on the journal's website. A resource for finding journals' instructions to authors is the website Instructions to Authors in the Health Sciences (http://mulford.utoledo.edu/instr/), from the Mulford Health Science Library at the University of Toledo (in Toledo, Ohio). This website provides links to instructions from more than 6,000 journals.

In guiding authors, medical editors sometimes suggest online resources on writing. One geared specifically to authors of medical journal articles is the Clinical Chemistry *Guide to Scientific Writing* (Annesley and Derish 2010–2011). Consisting of 14 articles from the journal *Clinical Chemistry*, this guide is essentially a free online textbook on writing articles for medical journals. Another resource that can be worth suggesting is Academic Phrasebank (https://www.phrasebank.manchester.ac.uk/), which lists phrases that can help convey given types of content in respective parts of journal articles. Websites of university writing centers also can be useful to recommend. These websites, which commonly are openly accessible, tend to include guidance on grammar, punctuation, and much more. Examples of writing center websites with much to offer are those of the Purdue University Online Writing Lab (OWL; https://owl.purdue.edu/owl/purdue_owl.html) and the Texas A&M University Writing Center (https://writingcenter.tamu.edu/). All these author-oriented websites can be instructive to editors as well.

Other websites that can be useful to bookmark include that of the EQUATOR (**E**nhancing the **QUA**lity and **T**ransparency **O**f health **R**esearch) Network (https://www.equator-network.org/), which provides links to guidelines for journal articles presenting types of medical research, and that of COPE (the Committee on Publication Ethics; https://publicationethics.org), which provides guidance on ethics in scholarly publication. Such resources will be discussed in the parts of this book on the respective topics.

Additional resources that can be worth bookmarking include the Copyeditors' Knowledge Base (https://www.kokedit.com/ckb.php) from longtime medical editor Katharine O'Moore-Klopf; among its components are one on editing tools and one on education and certification. The "Critical Tools for Medical Editing" page (https://dragonflyeditorial.com/resources/guide-to-medical-editing/) on the website of Dragonfly Editorial can be helpful as well.

Social media also can help medical editors find information for their work; stay more generally informed about the field; share knowledge, resources, and views; and gain or maintain visibility. In keeping with previous discussion, professional organizations' email discussion lists, online forums, Facebook groups, blogs, and other social media can be valuable resources. Examples of other resources to consider include the email discussion list Copyediting-L (see https://www.copyediting-l.info/) and its archive, the Medical Editors group on Facebook, and relevant groups and individuals on LinkedIn.

Tools for Your Office

As a medical editor, you will need access to (and competence with) basic office tools such as word-processing programs. You may also want or need other such tools, depending on the scope of your work and your work style. If you work in an editorial office, most or all of the tools probably will be provided. However, if you do mainly freelance work, you probably will need to obtain them yourself.

Much of what medical editors edit arrives in Microsoft Word and is edited in this program. Thus, you should be adept with Word. In particular, you need skill with the Track Changes feature, which shows the edits and comments made on a manuscript and so is widely used in editing. You may also need or want to use other products in the Microsoft Office suite. For instance, if your work includes editing presentations, you probably will need PowerPoint. And the spreadsheet program Excel can, among other things, aid in keeping track of your work. For some medical editors, work may arrive in Google Docs. Therefore, adeptness with it also is of value.

As a medical editor, you typically will use Adobe Acrobat to read, create, and otherwise work with PDF files. Other Adobe products also may be relevant. For example, if your work includes editing photos and refining illustrations, you might use Photoshop and Illustrator. Likewise, if you are involved in page design, you may well work with InDesign. Also in the visual vein: Two resources that can aid in developing illustrations are NIH BIOART (https://bioart.niaid.nih.gov/), which contains free visuals in medicine and biomedical science, and BioRender (https://www.biorender.com), which has templates and icons.

Other programs can help in detecting and resolving errors and aberrations. These programs include grammar checkers (such as Grammarly), medical spellcheckers (such as that from Stedman's), the proofreading program PerfectIt, and plagiarism-checking software (such as iThenticate). It should be noted that these programs do not prove that problems exist. Rather, they identify items that their algorithms deem worthy of suspicion. The conscientious medical editor then checks whether there is indeed a problem and, if the program has posed a solution, determines whether that solution is appropriate. Human judgment is needed.

"Plagiarism checkers" just indicate the degree of duplication between the current document and the documents in its database. They do not prove whether the duplication constitutes plagiarism or, for example, just reflects extensive use of standard phrasing. In a relatively formulaic journal article, substantial overlap with wording of previous articles can be warranted. At the other extreme, sometimes—as with the use of a single line of poetry in a medical essay—even minor overlap can constitute plagiarism unless permission for use was obtained.

Even wrong "corrections" from tools such as grammar checkers can aid an editor. Sometimes the software errs because a sentence has an odd structure or because a word that can be either a noun or a verb is interpreted as one instead of the other. If the software "misread" the sentence, human readers might well do so, especially if they are in a hurry, have limited English proficiency, or are literal-minded. Thus, although the suggestions from the software may be nonsensical, they can flag a lack of clarity and so lead the editor to recast the sentence in a form not easily misread.

Among some medical editors, strong feelings exist about readability checkers, such as that underlying the "show readability statistics" option in Word. Detractors note that these checkers, which use formulas based on word length and sentence length, do not assess readability per se; indeed, gobbledygook consisting of short sentences with short words could erroneously be rated as highly readable. However, excessively long sentences and unwarranted use of long words often do make medical writing needlessly hard to understand. By indicating that a document might have such problems, readability checkers can alert editors that streamlining the writing may be advisable.

Sometimes a medical editor's duties include editing references. Reference management software can aid in that regard. Such software lets the author or other user establish a database of references to employ. It also allows the reference format to be specified. Thus, for example, if a reference list is formatted for a given journal but instead the paper will go to a journal requiring a different reference format, the software can change the formatting as needed. Many medical researchers use the proprietary reference management software called EndNote. Another proprietary reference manager is RefWorks. Free software for reference management also is available; popular options include Mendeley and Zotero.

Electronic tools that have more recently emerged include those employing artificial intelligence (AI). Some medical researchers use AI tools such as ChatGPT to help them write articles that are clearer, more readable, and mechanically sounder than otherwise would be feasible for them. In particular, many authors for whom English is not a native language have found AI tools helpful in this regard (Sebastian and Baron 2024). Authors' use of such tools can decrease the number of mechanical problems for editors to correct and reduce the amount of querying needed. However, they do not eliminate the need for medical editors, who still must evaluate and refine the writing produced. Sometimes medical editors themselves can find AI tools helpful, for example in generating possible titles for a piece. The use of AI in medical writing and editing is evolving, and so the main advice is to keep informed. Sources of timely, suitably targeted information include professional societies such as the Council of Science Editors and the American Medical Writers Association, which have been keeping editors and others versed in this realm through their periodicals, webinars, and conferences.

As helpful as electronic tools can be, physical tools remain worth considering. Printing out a manuscript—or an especially challenging part thereof—can facilitate understanding and editing. Some medical editors like to do their initial editing on paper, for example using a favorite type of mechanical pencil or a pen with ink of a favorite color. Some of us like to use physical calendars and planners, instead of or in addition to electronic versions, to keep track of our work. And handwritten notes to thank or congratulate authors or others can add a memorable personal touch.

What about the physical setup? If you are employed in an editorial office, the setup might well be largely determined, though you may be able to adapt it. If you work remotely or do freelance work, you probably have more choice. And there is no single right choice. Are you someone needing an ergonomic setup to feel well and work well, or are you most comfortable at your kitchen table or in your favorite corner of the coffee shop? Do you like to have music playing, do you want silence, or do you fall somewhere in between? Do you work best with your dog at your feet or your cat at the keyboard, or would even a houseplant get you wheezing? Or do you become so engrossed in your editing that you're oblivious to your surroundings? Do what works for you.

Your Colleagues

Humans too can be tremendously helpful resources for medical editors. The medical editing community tends to be highly collegial, and members often serve as resources for each other. Do not hesitate to consult colleagues near or far. Most are glad, and even honored, to be consulted. Reach out to individuals whose knowledge and judgment you respect, or pose questions in email discussion lists or online forums. As well as conferring with fellow medical editors, consider consulting colleagues in allied fields—for example, science editors more generally, writing instructors, and medical librarians. And be willing to reciprocate, both by responding to requests and by taking the initiative to share. By helping each other, we can all promote excellence in medical editing.

Key Points

- Key resources for medical editors include style manuals, such as the *AMA Manual of Style*, and medical dictionaries.
- Other books useful to medical editors include medical books and articles, books on medical writing, and *The Copyeditor's Handbook*.
- Organizations in science editing and related fields have much to offer medical editors. To benefit most from these organizations, become actively involved.
- Journals' instructions to authors are an important resource for medical editors editing journal articles.

- College and university courses, non-degree certificate programs, open and other online courses, internships, and professional organizations' educational offerings can help medical editors develop, maintain, and update their knowledge and skills.
- Key online resources include PubMed for searching the medical literature.
- Fellow medical editors can be a tremendously helpful resource.

· 3 ·
Approaching an Editing Project

Before even touching a manuscript, a medical editor needs context. For example: What is the purpose of the piece of writing? What are the intended audience and venue? At what stage is the manuscript? What will happen after the current editing? What intensity of editing is appropriate? What are the authors' expectations? This chapter will both describe where medical editing fits in and discuss obtaining needed context when embarking on an editing project. It also will discuss possible orders in which to approach editing tasks.

Understanding the Context: The Writing and Editing Processes

Most medical writing undergoes multiple rounds of revision, and medical editors may take part in one or more of them. Also, most medical writing has multiple authors, with one author taking the lead and serving as the point of contact for editors. Understanding the usual processes for common types of medical writing, such as journal articles and grant proposals, can orient medical editors. Likewise, realizing that editorial processes can differ among types of medical writing can be helpful. For example, whereas a journal article may undergo repeated rounds of revision over months, in close consultation with the author, a news article for a website may be edited in literally minutes, without consulting the author and with much less attention to detail. Similarly, editorial processes and interactions can differ in other editorial contexts, such as those for books, regulatory documents, or medical licensing examinations. Awareness that such differences exist can aid medical editors who edit more than one type of document or who move to new editorial roles.

JOURNAL ARTICLES

Journal articles are central to medical communication, and various editors take part in their preparation and publication. Medical editors also consult journal articles in their work, and some edit news stories and news releases based on such articles. Thus, knowing how journal articles are produced and published can benefit medical editors. This process is summarized in the accompanying table.

In medicine, journal articles end up serving two main functions. The primary function is to share information, especially about findings of new medical research. Journal articles also serve as evidence of scholarly achievement, for example when health professionals and medical scientists are being considered for promotion. The resulting dynamics can affect how authors approach writing and publication and how they interact with medical editors in their institutions and at journals.

In most medical journals, the main articles report new research that the authors have done. Some medical journals also include other types of articles, such as reports of noteworthy cases, review articles summarizing knowledge on a topic, or commentary. Typically, the author listed first is the person who took the lead in the research and gets most credit, and the remaining authors are the other individuals with substantial intellectual contributions to the research. By tradition, commonly the senior researcher who heads the laboratory or research group is listed last. Exactly whom to list as authors, and in which order, can sometimes be a source of uncertainty and even contention. One widely recognized set of authorship criteria in medical fields is that of the International Committee of Medical Journal Editors. These criteria are posted at https://www.icmje.org/recommendations/browse/roles-and-responsibilities/defining-the-role-of-authors-and-contributors.html (International Committee of Medical Journal Editors, n.d.).

Early on, authors should consider where to submit their paper. Ideally, they should prepare a ranked list, as the first-choice journal might not accept the paper. Selecting a first-choice target journal and writing the paper accordingly, rather than writing a generic paper and then deciding on a journal, has two main benefits. First, it facilitates gearing the paper to the focus and audience of the chosen journal; for example, a paper about research on an infectious disease should be geared somewhat differently for a general scientific journal, a general medical journal, a journal for infectious-disease clinicians, and a microbiology journal. Second, having a specific journal in mind helps ensure that its requirements, such as those for format and length, are met. Gearing the manuscript to the journal from the start tends to work better than revamping a generic paper to suit it. If authors have access to an *author's editor* (an editor working with authors to help prepare papers for submission), the author's editor may help in choosing a journal, ensuring that its guidelines are followed, and ensuring that the paper suits the journal's focus and readership.

Sometimes the first-listed author drafts the entire article, and sometimes different authors draft different parts. In either case, the other authors should then provide feedback. The draft is then revised once or more before submission to a journal. Along the way—perhaps most commonly when the paper is nearly ready for submission—an author's editor may edit the paper. Usually, the lead author serves as the point of contact with this editor. The authors can accept, reject, or modify the revisions provided by the author's editor.

The *manuscript* (unpublished paper) is then submitted to the journal, commonly through an online portal. One author—commonly the first—serves as the *corresponding author* (point of contact for communications with the journal and, if the paper is published, point of contact for readers with questions about the paper). In some settings, an author's editor helps with submission. Some journals require that a cover letter accompany the paper. An author's editor may help in ensuring that the cover letter includes all required content and is effectively written.

Once the manuscript arrives, one or more people at or associated with the journal screen it to decide whether it merits further evaluation. At some medical journals, this screening is just to see whether the subject falls within the journal's scope (rather than, say, being on basic science if the journal is clinical) and whether the manuscript is generally in proper format (rather than, say, being twice the maximum allowed length). Some other journals—especially those that are highly selective—are more stringent in their screening. If the research clearly does not meet the journal's standards or the screeners deem the research lacking in suf-

Writing and Publishing a Journal Article: Editors and Their Contributions

STAGE	ACTIVITY	EDITORIAL INVOLVEMENT
Writing and Revision ↓	Authors write and revise the paper.	*Author's editor* (at the authors' institution or freelance) may help the authors refine the paper and help ensure it follows the journal's instructions.
Submission of Paper ↓	Author submits the paper, commonly through an online portal.	*Author's editor* or *editorial assistant* may help with the submission process.
Tracking of Paper ↓	Journal keeps track of the paper's status throughout review and publication.	*Managing editor* and others keep track of the paper, commonly through an electronic tracking system.
Screening by the Journal ↓	Journal screens paper to decide whether it qualifies for further review.	*Editorial assistant* or other staffer may screen paper to see if it meets basic requirements (for example, regarding completeness and length). *Editor-in-chief* or other *scientific editor* may briefly review the paper to see whether its quality seems to merit peer review.
Peer Review ↓	Experts in the authors' field evaluate the paper, mainly for quality of content.	*Editor-in-chief* or other *scientific editors* identify potential peer reviewers. *Managing editor* or other staff member arranges for the peer review.
Editorial Decision ↓	Based on the peer reviewers' assessments, the journal's own evaluation of the paper, and the journal's priorities and constraints, the journal decides whether to accept the paper as is (a rare occurrence), accept the paper if requested revisions are made, reconsider the paper if requested revisions are made, or reject the paper.	*Editor-in-chief* and/or *other scientific editors* (for example, associate editors) decide whether to accept the paper. One of the above prepares a letter informing the authors of the decision and (if relevant) listing requested revisions. Normally, feedback from the peer reviewers accompanies the letter.
Revision ↓	If the paper has not been rejected, the author revises it in keeping with the journal's requests, prepares a response to the requests, and submits a revised manuscript. The response may include rebuttals to some requests.	*Author's editor* (at the authors' institution or freelance) may help the authors to interpret the journal's requests, to make requested revisions, and to prepare the response, including any rebuttals.

STAGE	ACTIVITY	EDITORIAL INVOLVEMENT
Final Approval ↓	If the journal deems the paper suitably revised, it accepts the paper, and the remaining steps ensue.	*Editor-in-chief* and/or other *scientific editors* decide whether the paper has been suitably revised and thus whether to accept it, to reject it, or to request further revision.
Transition to Production ↓	The paper is scheduled for publication and enters the publication process.	Depending on the size and structure of the journal, individuals such as a *managing editor* and a *production editor* may be involved.
Manuscript Editing ↓	The accepted manuscript is edited to suit the journal.	*Manuscript editor* edits the manuscript. At some journals, the manuscript undergoes only *copyediting* (for mechanics, and for compliance with the journal's style and format). At other journals, the manuscript also receives *substantive editing*. *Manuscript editor* may be a journal staff member, a freelancer, or an employee of an editing company.
Review of Edited Manuscript ↓	One or more of the authors review the edited manuscript, mainly to ensure that the intended meaning has been retained.	*Author's editor* may assist with the review.
Production of Proofs ↓	The journal designs the pages of the article as they are to appear in the journal.	*Design staff* at or hired by the journal lays out the pages.
Review of Proofs ↓	The author(s) and others review the page proofs for accuracy.	*Editorial staff members* at the journal also review the proofs. *Author's editor* may help the author(s) review the proofs.
Publication ↓	The paper appears in the journal—typically either online only or both online and in print. At some journals, the paper also is posted online at one or more earlier stages.	*Various editors* and the authors have much to celebrate.
Publicity	In some instances, the paper is publicized through news releases, social media, or both. Also, journalists may report on the paper.	*Editors* at the journal or the authors' institution may edit the news release and social media posts. *Editors* in various media may edit resulting stories.

Note: This table presents an overall prototype of the process. At some journals, the process differs somewhat in some regards.

ficient novelty or otherwise unexciting, the paper may be returned to the authors without further review. Return at this point is sometimes termed a "desk reject." The authors can then submit the paper to another journal. Of course, the paper should first be revised to suit the new journal. An author's editor can help in that regard.

If a paper passes the initial screening, an editor at the journal sends the paper for *peer review*—in other words, evaluation by fellow experts in the authors' field. The number of peer reviewers can depend on the journal's norms and the nature of the paper; a paper reporting interdisciplinary research may need more reviewers than a paper in a narrow research area. Commonly, the paper goes to two to four reviewers. Time allotted for the reviews varies among journals and sometimes is reduced if the research seems especially timely (for instance, because it regards a current outbreak of a disease). Many journals give reviewers between two and four weeks to complete reviews.

The main role of the *peer reviewers* (sometimes termed *referees*) is to advise the journal editor on whether to publish the research. Thus, the key focus is on content, not writing style. Accordingly, peer reviewers commonly are asked to address questions such as the following: Does the research address an important question? Does the research show originality? Have appropriate research methods been used? Do the results seem plausible? Are the conclusions consistent with the results? Overall, is the paper well crafted? Journals generally have reviewers submit their reviews in two parts. One part, which is confidential to the journal editors, addresses questions such as those above and includes a recommendation about whether to publish the paper. The other part, which goes both to the journal's editors and to the paper's authors, presents constructive criticism of the paper. Commonly, it begins by noting the paper's overall strengths and limitations and then presents line-by-line comments, especially suggestions. Sometimes, if a paper seems promising, the editor also sends it to a statistical reviewer to assess more thoroughly whether the study design and statistical analyses are sound.

After reading the paper and receiving the peer reviews, the editor (or group of editors) at the journal decides how to proceed. A common misconception is that editors just tally reviewers' "votes." However, the process is more complex. The decision whether to publish a given paper depends on multiple factors, including not only the reviewers' bottom-line recommendations but also such items as the reasons stated for those recommendations, the amount of room in the journal, the balance of subject matter in the journal, the perceived interest to readers, and—yes—the quality of the writing (and thus the amount of revision likely to be needed to make the paper publishable). Very rarely, an editor of a medical journal may decide to accept a paper entirely as is. Normally, if a paper is accepted, the acceptance is contingent on making requested revisions. In some other instances, a journal does not accept the paper but expresses willingness to reconsider it if the authors make the requested changes (such as including more information so the research can be evaluated more thoroughly or even doing additional experiments). The authors can then decide whether to pursue this option or submit the paper elsewhere. Or the journal may decide not to publish the paper. At prominent, highly competitive journals—which receive many more papers than they can publish—such rejection is common. Often, papers that are basically sound but not deemed of high enough priority can find good homes in journals that are more specialized.

Regardless of the decision, the authors normally receive the peer reviewers' comments. These comments can both aid in refining the current paper and prove instructive for future work. And whatever the journal's decision, an author's editor may be able to help the authors revise their paper for resubmission or for submission elsewhere.

After acceptance by a medical journal, a paper normally undergoes some editing before publication. (Some online journals, though, do not edit papers. Rather, if they deem a paper poorly written but otherwise acceptable, they require the authors to have it edited if it is to be published. In this situation, some journals identify editing companies to consider.) Sometimes, the editing of accepted papers is by manuscript editors on the journal's staff. In other instances, the journal engages freelance manuscript editors (sometimes including former journal staff members) or professional editing companies for this purpose. At many journals, editing at this stage tends to be relatively light, consisting mainly of editing for mechanics (such as grammar, spelling, and punctuation) and for consistency with the journal's style (such as regarding number format and reference format). At some journals with more resources, the editing tends to be more extensive, sometimes including reorganization, rewording, redrawing of figures, or other changes. After the editing, the author normally receives the edited manuscript to review, mainly to ensure that the intended meaning has been retained. If the manuscript editor has questions—for example about material that seems to be inconsistent, missing, or ambiguous—the author also may receive *queries* to answer.

Finally, there will be *proofs* (copies of the paper as it is to appear once published) to review and, if necessary, correct. The corresponding author receives the proofs, commonly as PDF files. One or more of the authors should then review them—for example, to ensure that images are properly oriented and that glitches in the text have not arisen during typesetting and design. One or more editors or proofreaders associated with the journal review the proofs as well. If the authors have worked with an author's editor, the author's editor can be a helpful extra set of eyes. Journals typically give authors relatively little time (for example, 48 or 72 hours) to review the proofs; authors should plan accordingly.

A note: In recent years, increasing numbers of medical authors have posted their articles online, as *preprints* in *preprint servers*, before submitting them to journals or instead of doing so. An author's editor can help ensure that such articles are readable and otherwise sound. Such an editor also can help refine such articles for later journal submission.

GRANT PROPOSALS

In addition to writing journal articles, medical authors may prepare a variety of other materials, such as grant proposals, books and book chapters, submissions to regulatory agencies, and materials for general readerships. Medical editors may assist with each and so can benefit from knowing the processes these writings undergo.

In academic settings, funding to conduct biomedical research generally comes from grants. Some of the largest, most competitive, and most prestigious of these grants come from US government agencies, especially the National Institutes of Health (NIH). Other sources of research grants include private foundations, some of which have large funding programs. In addition, some universities and other research institutions have internal grants available to their researchers.

To be considered for a grant, researchers must submit a *proposal*, or *grant application*. Typically, major parts of the proposal include background on the research topic and its importance, a statement of one or more hypotheses or research questions, a plan for the research, information about the researchers (usually in the form of curricula vitae or specifically formatted biosketches), and a proposed budget. Funders of major grants tend to have detailed instructions to follow and strict deadlines for proposal submission, and an application for a major grant can be a complex document running many pages. Some smaller funders seek shorter, simpler proposals and have more flexibility. Preparing a major grant proposal can take several months.

Typically, one researcher, termed the *principal investigator*, or *PI*, takes the lead in writing and submitting the proposal. Other members of the proposed research team, who may be at the PI's institution or elsewhere, may contribute content and help refine the proposal. In addition, specialized staff may help with aspects such as preparing the budget and obtaining needed approvals from administrators at the involved institution(s). An editor may assist as well. Ideally, the editor's involvement should begin early. The editor may then help in planning the content and structure of the proposal, gathering materials from participants, and ensuring that all requirements are met, in addition to polishing the text (a worthwhile endeavor only if the proposal is otherwise sound).

Such polishing can be important, so the proposal is clear, readable, and persuasive and conveys competence. A reason: Like journal manuscripts, proposals normally undergo peer review. For example, at NIH they are reviewed by committees, called *study sections*, consisting of researchers with expertise in the research area of the proposal. These peer reviewers, who come from various institutions, typically are prominent researchers with many other demands on their time and many proposals to review. Therefore, proposals that are hard to follow face a disadvantage. For some funding sources, reviewers also include laypeople committed to the source's mission. In this case, the writing must also be clear to nonspecialists. Competition for grants from governmental and many other funding sources is high, with only a small proportion of proposals funded. Good editing may give a proposal the needed edge. Indeed, with so much at stake, freelance editing of grant proposals tends to command higher rates than some other areas of freelance medical editing.

Some funding sources share peer reviewers' feedback with the grant applicant. If a proposal showed promise but the research was not funded, staff at the funding agency may suggest that the applicant consider revising the proposal and reapplying. An editor can assist the applicant in assimilating the feedback and strengthening the proposal. Similarly, at various stages editors can assist in applying for grants for non-research initiatives, such as training programs and outreach programs.

BOOKS

Another category of proposal is that for a book. Before writing a medically related book, the usual procedure is to submit a proposal for it to one or more publishers, such as commercial publishing companies or university presses. The author sometimes contacts the publisher beforehand, to assess potential interest. In addition, acquisitions editors at publishers sometimes invite medical experts to submit proposals. A book proposal typically includes a cover letter, an annotated table of contents, a sample chapter, a curriculum vitae or resume, and a description of the market for the book. A freelance editor or an editor at the proposer's institution may aid in developing or refining the book proposal.

After the book proposal arrives, staff at the publisher screen it to see whether it might be suitable. If it passes the screening, it receives more thorough assessment, often including peer review and an analysis of financial viability. If all seems favorable, the proposer may receive an advance contract for the book. Then the bulk of the writing begins. Sometimes, for a single-authored book, the author may enlist an editor to help in developing the manuscript or in refining it before submission. If the book will be multiauthored, with chapters by various experts, the proposer may enlist an editor to help manage the project and otherwise assist.

Once the manuscript is submitted, staff at the publisher review it. Especially if the publisher is a university press or scholarly commercial publisher, the manuscript may undergo peer review. If the feedback is favorable overall, the acquisitions editor then conveys to the author any suggestions (or requirements) for revision. In making revisions, authors sometimes work with author's editors. Once the publisher deems the manuscript suitably revised, it accepts the manuscript. (Not all book manuscripts reach this stage—but guidance from internal and external editors can help ensure that a manuscript does so.) At university presses, final acceptance typically requires approval by a faculty committee.

The accepted manuscript then enters production, under supervision of a production editor. Sometimes production is overseen solely in-house; in other instances, coordination of aspects of production is outsourced. Major aspects of book production include copyediting the manuscript, either by editors on the publisher's staff or by freelance editors (such as those specializing in medical editing). Other aspects of production include cover design, page design, indexing, and printing. Editors also edit marketing materials for the book.

AND MORE

Medical editors also help to develop and refine magazine articles, other health-related writings for general readerships, regulatory and other materials from medically related corporations, and more. Here too, knowing the processes helps in identifying opportunities and working effectively.

A magazine may include articles by magazine staff members, freelance writers, or both. Editors at magazines work with staff writers to decide on article topics. Likewise, they may invite freelance writers to prepare articles on given topics; perhaps more commonly, freelance writers submit proposals, known as *query letters* or *pitches*, for articles they wish to write, and editors decide whether to accept them. For both staffers and freelancers, an editor may help shape the article from early on, for example by helping to define its scope and by recommending people to interview and other information sources to consult. Once the article is submitted, the editor may suggest revisions. Either the same editor, another editor on the staff, or a freelance editor will copyedit the article before posting or printing. At various stages of the process, an editor knowledgeable about medical content, medical information sources, and the presentation of medical information can help ensure that articles are informative, accurate, and suitably crafted.

Pharmaceutical, biotechnology, and medical device companies produce a wide variety of documents, for a wide variety of audiences—including regulatory agencies, health professionals, the media, patients, and other members of the general public. Perhaps most distinctive are the regulatory documents that government agencies such as the US Food and Drug Administration require for use in determining whether to approve products such as drugs. These documents, which can be very lengthy, must meet strict requirements for content and format. To prepare and refine these documents, medical writers and editors—either on staff or freelance—work with researchers, statisticians, and others at or associated with the company.

Government agencies, such as the US National Institutes of Health, produce a variety of informational materials for the general public and others. Some of these materials are by subject-matter specialists such as physicians and scientists, and others are by medical writers. The materials must undergo a clearance process, in which they are reviewed and approved at various administrative levels. As well as doing the initial editing, a medical editor may be responsible for navigating the clearance process and helping to make revisions that reviewers require. Similarly, outside of government, at health-related organizations such as those concerned with specific diseases, medical editors may both edit documents and manage their approval for release.

In short, where there is writing about medicine, there is (or should be) editing too. Knowing the writing process for a given type of document or in a given context, and knowing where editing fits in, can help a medical editor to function well.

Recognizing Differences Between Literary and Medical Editing

Knowing where medical editing fits in and approaching a writing project accordingly also can entail understanding differences between literary and medical editing. For editors accustomed mainly to norms for literary writing, some expectations for medical editing can seem surprising or downright wrong. Awareness of the following differences can aid in approaching medical writing—and medical authors—appropriately.

- *Elaboration versus conciseness*: Editors often encourage literary authors to elaborate on what they have said. In medical writing, however, conciseness is valued, to efficiently use readers' time and the available space. Thus, medical editing commonly includes condensing text rather than encouraging authors to expand it.
- *Variation versus consistency in wording*: In literary contexts, authors often are urged to vary their wording. In medical writing, however, consistency in wording is favored, to avoid ambiguity and promote cohesiveness. If medical authors did a study in mice, they generally should keep referring to them as *mice*—not add variety by also saying *rodents*, *animals*, *creatures*, *organisms*, and *beings*.
- *Connotation versus denotation*: In literary work, multiple levels of meaning, and openness to multiple interpretations, can be highly desirable. In medical writing, however, all readers should come away with the same single message—such as exactly how a study was

performed, exactly what findings were obtained, or exactly what guidelines to follow in treatment. Medical writing should be edited accordingly.

- *Visibility versus invisibility of the writing*: Oftentimes, literary writing should be apparent as writing. It can be desirable for readers to notice the writing style and to remark on the item's crafting. In contrast, medical writing generally should be "invisible": Readers should be able to grasp the content without even noticing the writing. Medical editing should strive to promote such effortless access.
- *The author's source of pride: the written piece versus the research*: For literary authors, the written product tends to be a source of pride. For medical authors, however, the main pride tends to lie in the research being reported. Accordingly, author-editor dynamics may differ. A literary author may be much more sensitive to proposed changes in wording; many medical authors care less about nuances of language but may focus more on sharing their work widely and rapidly and in a prestigious venue.
- *Location on the "therapist-to-accountant spectrum"*: Literary writing and the production thereof can be highly personal, and some literary editors, such as Maxwell Perkins (Berg 1978), have served as counselors and confidants and more. Interactions between medical authors and those editing their writing, though typically cordial, tend to remain more formal and focused. To use an image from health care: Though attentive to authors' state of mind, the medical editor may be less a psychiatrist and more a primary care practitioner, medical subspecialist, or surgeon.

Considering the Stage of the Manuscript—and of the Author

Regardless of the type of manuscript, how to approach the writing as an editor depends in part on its stage of development. It also can depend somewhat on the author's stage of familiarity with writing and editing.

GEARING THE EDITING TO THE STAGE OF THE MANUSCRIPT

Early in the writing process—when the writer has prepared a rough draft or is planning the document—a medical editor can most usefully focus on overall content and organization. Does the structure comply with requirements and conventions for the type of document? Within given sections, is the flow of ideas logical and in keeping with expectations in the field? Do any major types of content seem to be missing? Do any chunks of content seem superfluous? At this stage, little point exists in polishing language or ensuring that every reference is perfectly formatted; after all, some of the text and references might not even appear in later versions. However, if repeated copyeditorial problems—such as a term used incorrectly many times or an error in formatting throughout—are noticed, now is a good time to alert the writer to correct the problem and avoid perpetuating it.

As the writing approaches submission, editing should become more granular. For example, grammar and spelling should be checked. Ditto for usage of medical and other terms. And ditto for clarity. If the document is to follow a particular style—such as AMA style for a journal article or AP style for a news release—now is the time to check for compliance with that style. Likewise, if a journal, granting agency, or other recipient has specific requirements for submission, now is a time to double-check for consistency with them. If the editor also was asked to do deeper editing—such as making the wording more concise, improving flow, and checking logic—now is also the time for such tasks.

However, now is not a time to dwell at length on details such as the format for an obscure type of reference. The rationale? The goal of pre-submission editing is to prepare the document to sail successfully through the next stage. For example, a journal submission should be clear, readable, and reasonably polished—so the initial impression on editors and peer reviewers will be of professionalism, so the journal can readily screen the submission, and so peer reviewers can easily understand the submission and accurately evaluate its content. Similarly, editing should help ensure that a grant proposal is written such that peer reviewers can readily judge the merits of what is being proposed. In short, in pre-submission editing, the key goal is to yield a submission excellently suited for evaluation based on its content, without distraction or misinterpretation because of unclear or sloppy writing. An article or proposal is unlikely indeed to be rejected because a hyphen should have been a dash (yes, there's a difference!) or because part of a reference that should have been italicized wasn't. Yes, be careful about such items even at this stage. But no need to agonize at length about them. Doing so is an inefficient use of your time—and a poor use of the resources of whoever is paying for the work.

Definitive attention to such details normally follows acceptance for publication. For example, a journal may ask the author of an accepted manuscript to resolve inconsistencies with the journal's reference style—and the author may, in turn, ask an author's editor for help in such regards. And a journal or book publisher may perform, or obtain from a contractor, final editing of the manuscript, including thorough editing for consistency with the publisher's style and format.

Medical editors also may do *proofreading*—the final checking of writing for typographical and related errors. An edited manuscript should be proofread before submission. Likewise, the proofs of an article or book must be proofread. Examples of items to look for when proofreading include typographical errors that were missed during editing or introduced during typesetting (for example, Greek letters that electronic gremlins converted to squiggles); mechanical errors (such as problems with subject-verb agreement) and style errors (such as absent serial commas) that were missed during editing; and, in the case of a page proof, page-layout problems (such as incorrect placement of figures and tables or awkward spacing of text). Traditionally, proofreaders' corrections have been made on hard copy, using proofreading symbols. Today, much proofreading is done electronically, for example by using Adobe Acrobat to indicate corrections on proofs that are in PDF. Technically, proofreading is not part of editing. But proofreading skills are a useful part of a medical editor's toolbox. And medical editors should be conversant enough with proofreading to know how it fits in and how to work well with proofreaders. Also, a job consisting largely of medical proofreading can be a good way to break into medical editing. Sources of guidance on proofreading include style manuals such as the *AMA Manual of Style* (AMA Manual of Style Committee 2020) and *The Chicago Manual of Style* (University of Chicago Press Editorial Staff 2024), as well as books specifically on proofreading. In addition, workshops and other resources on proofreading are available through organizations such as the American Medical Writers Association.

GEARING THE EDITING TO THE STAGE OF THE AUTHOR

The nature of editing also can depend on the author's career stage. For early-career authors (such as students, residents, and postdoctoral fellows), the most productive approach can be "educational editing." Such editing is intended both to improve the current piece of writing and to help the author develop knowledge and skills that can improve future writing. In educational editing, an editor (or a faculty mentor) provides explanations more thorough than those in typical author's editing. These explanations may include comments (commonly presented in Track Changes) saying why particular changes in grammar, punctuation, capitalization, or word usage were made and advising the author to follow these norms in the future. Similarly, when making wording more concise and direct, the editor may explain to the early-career author the value of writing readably rather than trying to sound scholarly—and may encourage the author to strive for such accessibility. If a manuscript has repeated problems of the same type, the editor may remedy the first instance or two and then ask the early-career author to remedy the remaining instances. Making these remaining corrections and revisions can reinforce the early-career author's learning and make efficient use of the editor's time. Similarly, in returning an edited manuscript to an early-career author, an editor may provide a cover note that is longer and more explanatory than one that would accompany an edited manuscript being returned to a more established author.

For authors later in their careers, a major goal of the editing may be to save the author time. Such authors may be overwhelmed with duties in clinic, laboratory, classroom, and more, and so they may lack the time to make their writing achieve its potential. An editor may be able to devote that time and thus improve and increase the author's output. Unless such an author so requests, the editing is unlikely to have an explicit educational component. Rare is the editor who would burden the typical chief of neurosurgery with an explanation of restrictive versus nonrestrictive clauses.

Deciding on Levels of Editing

Editing isn't editing isn't editing. Rather, different intensities of editing exist. Before starting to edit a manuscript, find out what intensity of editing the author or publisher expects, look at the manuscript to assess what intensity of editing seems appropriate, or both. Sometimes, once an editing project is underway, you may find that a different intensity is more suitable, and so expectations may need to be revised. Nonetheless, having some sense of the wanted or needed intensity can be helpful from the start—lest a recipient wanting a deep review of a document be disappointed to find only mechanical corrections, or lest a recipient expecting only mechanical corrections be shocked to find that a document has also been reorganized, condensed, and peppered with queries about content.

In the field of editing, intensities of editing traditionally are called *levels of editing*. These levels are *light*, *medium*, and *heavy*.

- *Light editing* is relatively superficial editing. It entails correcting mechanical errors, such as those in grammar, spelling, punctuation, and word usage. It also entails correcting deviations from the requested style. For example, if a manuscript is to be in AMA style, in which the serial comma is required, light editing would include adding such commas where they are missing.
- *Medium editing* includes, in addition to the items entailed in light editing, revision of the text for readability. Thus, for example, it includes making wordy writing more concise. It also includes recasting awkward sentences to read more smoothly.
- *Heavy editing* includes the items in light and medium editing but also goes more deeply, addressing content and organization. Thus, revisions that are made or suggested in heavy editing may include adding content, deleting content, reorganizing the document or parts of it, checking items for accuracy, making reasoning sounder or clearer, and rewriting passages.

Despite use of the terms *light*, *medium*, and *heavy*, a continuum exists, rather than three discrete categories. Indeed, different editors sometimes define the borders between levels somewhat differently. What's important is not which category the editing is said to fall into but rather that the editing is an appropriate intensity. Also, "levels of editing" is sometimes misconstrued as indicating the number of revisions—rather than types of revisions—made. However, editing may include multiple corrections per sentence but still be light editing if all the corrections are of mechanical errors. Or the editing may consist of few changes overall but still be heavy editing if the changes regard content or organization.

The range of levels of editing can be likened to that of medical or dental interventions. At one extreme, some such interventions—though sometimes extensive—are cosmetic. At the other extreme, some are vital, though they may be small in scope. The light verse at the beginning of this book (Gastel 1993) captures this analogy.

Two concepts related to levels of editing are *microediting* (Churchill 2001) versus *macroediting* (Churchill, Tacker, and Porcher 2001) and *copyediting* versus *substantive editing*. *Microediting* is editing for detail, largely at the sentence or paragraph level or below; it corresponds to light or medium editing. *Macroediting* is big-picture editing, focusing mainly on overall content and organization. Sometimes *copyediting* is used as a synonym for manuscript editing in general. In its narrow sense, though, *copyediting* refers to light or medium editing, including correction of mechanical errors and editing for consistency with the requested style. In contrast, *substantive editing* focuses on the substance of the writing and so is concerned largely with content and organization. By the way, the *copy* in *copyediting* does not mean copy in the sense of duplication; rather, it refers to *copy* meaning text for publication.

Communicating About Expectations

To an editor of medical writing, it may be obvious why the writing will be edited and what path the manuscript will take once the author provides it. To an author, not necessarily so. Authors may have little sense of the publication process. They also may mistakenly view editors as condescending, judgmental appliers of arbitrary rules. (Alas, they may have encountered editors who fit this stereotype.) They may be generalizing from painful experiences having writing graded as students. They may think that editing is proofreading, or that proofreading is editing. They may think that authors with full English proficiency do not need editors. They may fear that the editing will introduce inaccuracies they will lack a chance to correct. Sadly, they may view the editor as the enemy.

So, in starting to work with an author, the first task often is to counter misconceptions and myths—and to show that the editor is the author's ally. Among items that may bear explanation to the author are the following:

- The editor and author share the common goals of ensuring that the writing communicates effectively with the reader, that the writing fulfills the criteria for acceptance, and that the author looks good.
- The editor brings a fresh eye (something that can benefit any piece of writing), expertise in written communication, familiarity with the expectations of the publication or other venue, acknowledgment that the author is the subject-matter expert, and a compassionate understanding of how difficult the writing process can be.
- If the writing already is in excellent condition, the editor may have

few changes to make, and thus review by an editor can provide reassurance. If the writing still could benefit from substantial revision, the editor can be seen as a consultant or coach. The writing remains the author's.

The author may be uncertain what the editing will consist of, or the author may have misconceptions in this regard. For *pre-submission editing* (*author's editing*), the editor and author should reach an overall understanding of the types of revisions to be made (the level of editing), while realizing that this understanding may evolve as the work does. The timetable should be discussed and, if relevant, the possibility of more than one round of editing mentioned. Especially when working with a given author for the first time, editing a short passage and then, if warranted, recalibrating expectations can help. Authors should be assured that they will receive their writing back and can then decide whether to keep, toss, or modify proposed revisions.

For author's editing, now can also be a good time to establish preferences or expectations regarding substance and working style. For example: Are there sections the author thinks could especially benefit from editing? Are there items that should not be changed—for example, wording that might seem strange but is standard in the field? Should queries be provided as comments in Track Changes, as is common? Or would the author like queries to be embedded in the text, perhaps in boldface or in colored type? Does the author like to know rationales for changes or not?

The author's editor also should obtain context. For example, for what journal or granting agency is the writing destined, and what are its instructions? Ideally, the author's editor should chat with the author before starting the editing. Helpful questions to ask may include "How did you come to do this work?" and "How, in brief, would you summarize this work?" As well as yielding useful information, such conversations can provide a sense of the author's personality and thus a sense of how best to interact. (For instance: Does this author seem to be a stickler who will want you to justify each suggestion, for example by quoting the style manual? Or does this author seem to be a laid-back soul who will need urging to answer queries?) Importantly, such a conversation can help show the author that you are a (reasonable) human being and are committed to the quality and integrity of the work. It also can help you see the author as a human being and approach the work accordingly.

For *publication editing*, such as editing accepted papers at a journal, there is less to explore with the author, as the type of editing to provide and the protocol for providing it tend to be relatively standardized. However, expectations still should be conveyed to the author, either by the manuscript editor or by another member of the staff. What kinds of edits will be made, and why? When will the author receive the edited text to review, and how long will the author have to respond? Providing such information early can ease authors' anxieties and facilitate publication.

Determining What to Do in What Order

So, you've now scoped out the editing project. Time to dig in. But how?

There's no one right answer. Different good editors favor somewhat different approaches, and the same editor may approach different projects differently. However, some basic considerations exist.

One basic consideration is backup. Be sure to keep a backup copy of the original manuscript. Also back up your editing electronically (or make sure your computer is set to automatically do so), lest hours (or more) of work be lost. In addition, have a system for labeling versions of files. For example, if I am editing a paper that Dr. Tom Vogel wrote about gout, perhaps the original file would be VogelGout2025July, my edited version would be VogelGout2025July_ed by BG, a revised version provided by Dr. Vogel after receiving the edits would be VogelGout2025July_ed by BG_rev by TV, and my final edited version would be VogelGout2025July_ed by BG_rev by TV_ed2 by BG.

As tempted as you may be to start refining the text right away, try to restrain yourself. Best practice generally is to read, or at least skim, the full document before starting to edit. Doing so lets you see the scope of the material, provides information that can aid in editing, and helps identify overall problems (if any) to address. It thus tends to prevent inefficiencies such as spending considerable time trying to discern what a given sentence means, only to find that a later passage provides clarification, or carefully wording a suggestion of something to add, only to find that the item is present elsewhere and perhaps just should be moved.

Different editors like to edit parts of a document such as a journal article in different orders. Some prefer to edit the reference list first. Some prefer to start with the figures and tables. Others prefer to begin at the beginning of the text. Regardless of the order, good editing requires more than one pass—because noticing everything in a single pass is nearly impossible, because the editing sometimes introduces problems that later need correction, and because some inconsistencies and other problems may not be apparent before immersion in the document as a whole. Also, some editors prefer to begin on the macro level, with overall content and organization, and then edit on the micro level, for mechanics such as grammar and punctuation; others, however, find that starting with mechanics helps them gain the close understanding that will best allow them to address macroscopic aspects. Often, a good tack is to alternate between macroediting and microediting, just as one might alternate between low power and high power of a microscope to best understand what appears on a microscope slide. Whatever the order, in the final pass the title and abstract generally should be reviewed last, to help ensure that these items are consistent with the rest of the document.

Finally, proofread the document. If you have been showing the editing in Track Changes, consider changing the setting to "No Markup" or the equivalent for this pass. This way, you may more easily notice (and correct) problems such as spacing errors introduced by the editing.

Congratulations on having approached the editing project well.

Key Points

- Knowing how medical journal articles are written and published can help medical editors function effectively. Ditto for knowing how grant proposals are prepared and reviewed and understanding the processes for other types of medical writing.
- Editing medical writing can differ from editing literary writing. For example, it favors conciseness rather than elaboration, consistency in wording rather than variation, denotation rather than connotation, and invisibility rather than visibility of the writing.
- In deciding how to approach an editing project, it can be helpful to consider the stage of development of the writing and the career stage of the author.
- Although proofreading is not editing per se, editors often are tasked with proofreading and so should be conversant with it.
- Different intensities of editing (commonly known as light, medium, and heavy editing) exist. It can be helpful to determine what intensity of editing is warranted and, if necessary, revise this assessment as the editing progresses.

- Authors sometimes have misconceptions about editing or lack knowledge about why and how it will take place. Therefore, initially explaining the reasons and plans can be advisable.
- Different editors approach aspects of editing a piece in different orders. Regardless of the order chosen, thorough editing requires reviewing the document more than once.

· 4 ·

Copyediting

EDITING FOR MECHANICS AND MORE

Much medical editing is *copyediting*—in other words, editing mainly to ensure that mechanics such as grammar and punctuation are correct and that the writing complies with the requested style and format. For medical documents, copyediting also includes helping to ensure that medical word usage is appropriate. Medical copyediting also can include editing tables and figures. So: Why copyedit? How should you correct errors, and when and how should you query about copyeditorial revisions? What are some medical aspects of usage to be alert for? What is meant by a publication's style, and how can you best comply with it? What are some basics of editing tables and figures, and how can you obtain more guidance in this regard? This chapter will address such questions.

Why Copyedit?

Why bother copyediting? Isn't it just a matter of correcting nitpicking details? Does it make any difference?

Medical copyediting can be important for a variety of reasons. The mechanics of writing are not just cosmetic. Mechanical errors can change meaning, hinder understanding, undermine confidence in the author, and cause downright embarrassment. (Just ask a former employee of the US Public Health Service who kept typing *pubic* instead of *public.*) Similarly, deviations from a publication's style can come across as sloppy and be confusing. And poorly edited tables and figures can be hard to follow. Indeed, readers may just give up on poorly copyedited tables, figures, and text. Hence, copyediting can play an important role in helping ensure that medical documents communicate effectively to their audiences.

Correcting and Querying

Copyediting text consists mainly of (1) correcting mechanical and style errors and (2) querying the author when a problem may exist but the editor needs more information to know how to proceed. How can you best do these items?

INDICATING EDITS

Traditionally, copyediting was done on paper, using conventional copyediting marks. A chart of such marks, with examples of their use, appears in *The Copyeditor's Handbook* (Einsohn and Schwartz 2019, 45–47). Charts of copyediting marks also can be readily found through searching online. Occasionally, writing still is edited this way: Editing by hand can be good practice for the beginning copyeditor, as using the proper mark requires understanding the nature of the change. Also, some experienced editors like to edit a document by hand before doing so onscreen, as they find they are more thorough in this way. For editing by hand, some editors like to use pencil, so they can correct their corrections. And some editors like to use green pen, to avoid the connotations of red pen. If corrections and queries that were made in pencil are to be given to the author, sending a scan or photocopy of the edited document, rather than the original, can be wise, lest the author simply erase some of the changes. And, of course, the editor should keep the original or a copy of the hand-edited document.

These days, medical copyediting usually is done electronically, using Track Changes. Corrections and proposed revisions appear in the text, and queries generally appear in comment bubbles. (See example in Appendix 1.) Corrections should be easy to read, to facilitate checking by authors, others (if any) such as editorial supervisors, and oneself. For instance, deleting an incorrectly spelled word and following it with the correctly spelled version tends to yield a more readable result than does changing individual letters. For example:

- Original version: opthamology and nuerosurgrey
- Awkwardly corrected version: ophthalmology and n~~u~~eurosurger~~e~~y
- Most readably corrected version: ~~opthamology~~ophthalmology and ~~nuerosurgrey~~neurosurgery

Similarly, deleting an unsuitable string of words and replacing it immediately afterward with the new version can work better than making piecemeal corrections. Consistently placing the revised word or words after the deleted material (rather than placing the new material beforehand or sometimes placing it one way and sometimes the other) is logical and can help make the editing easy to follow. Thus, for example, "~~opthamology~~ophthalmology and ~~nuerosurgrey~~neurosurgery" or "~~opthamology and nuerosurgrey~~ophthalmology and neurosurgery" is preferable to such options as "ophthalmology~~opthamology~~ and neurosurgery~~nuerosurgrey~~" and "~~opthamology~~ophthalmology and neurosurgery~~nuerosurgrey~~." Further advice appears in the two-article series "Author-Friendly Onscreen Editing" (Deming 2009b, 2009c) by Stephanie Deming, a longtime author's editor at the University of Texas MD Anderson Cancer Center.

QUERYING AUTHORS

In copyediting medical writing, you may find that information is missing, that content is inconsistent, or that an error seems to exist other than in mechanics or style. For example: A reference might be cited but not appear in the reference list. A number in the text may differ from the corresponding number in a table. Or the spelling of a name might seem highly implausible. Sometimes you can resolve the difficulty yourself, for example by checking a name in an authoritative directory. But often, to obtain the answer, you must ask the author of the piece you are editing. In other words, you need to query. You also should query if you are uncertain whether a revision you made has retained the intended meaning. (In substantive editing, which addresses content and organization in addition to mechanics and style, you might also query about additional types of items. For example, you might suggest adding or deleting information on a topic, reorganizing a passage, or clarifying reasoning.)

As noted, queries commonly appear as comments in Track Changes. If queries are handwritten on hard copy, they generally are written in the margin and are circled, to distinguish them from additions to the text. If a query is too lengthy to provide feasibly as a Track Changes comment or marginal note, or if it regards a general aspect of the document, a good option can be to provide the query in an accompanying document, such as a cover memo.

Queries should be polite yet concise. And, of course, they should be clear. The following are examples of some not-so-good queries and improved versions.

Overly vague query: "Is something missing here?"
Improved query: "A study by Castiglioni is noted here, but no reference is cited. Please add the appropriate reference."

Excessively wordy query: "The table states that 345 patients reported nausea, but the text says that 354 patients did so. Maybe the digits were just transposed, but of course I have no way of knowing which number, if either, is correct. I do realize that maybe the numbers are different for a good reason. If so, I think you should provide an explanation, lest the peer reviewers object to the difference in numbers or lest readers become confused. I look forward to receiving your reply."
Improved query: "The table states that 345 patients reported nausea, but the text says that 354 patients did so. Please resolve the discrepancy. Thanks!"

Impolite query: "Huh? Those numbers don't make sense."
Improved query: "Based on the data given, this percentage seems incorrect. Please check."

Impolite query: "Plagiarized! Don't you know it's unethical?"
Improved query: "This paragraph appears to be the same as in ____, which you cited. To avoid plagiarism, please present the information in your own words. I would be glad to help."

Query only when needed. If a change is a simple mechanical one, no need to flag it. Here are two examples of unnecessary queries.

Unnecessary query: "The list is alphabetical with one exception: The entry for Fraumeni precedes that for Fauci. Would you like to reverse the order?"
Solution: No query is needed here. Just go ahead and reverse the order.

Unnecessary query: "I italicized the genus and species here, as is standard and as was done elsewhere in this manuscript. OK?"

Solution: Again, no query is needed.

Sometimes, however, noting mechanical edits or style edits can be appropriate. For example, if an appropriate edit might mistakenly be viewed as introducing an error, queries such as the following can clarify the situation.

Example: The target journal uses British spellings (such as *paediatrics*), and so the text has been revised accordingly.

Example: I realize that in earlier editions of this book we lowercased *black* and *white* when referring to races. However, in keeping with updated guidance in the *AMA Manual of Style* and other stylebooks, these items have now been capitalized.

Likewise, if you are doing "educational editing," or if the author likes to know reasons for changes, queries presenting explanations can be in order.

Example from educational editing: Normally, names of disciplines should be lowercase unless part of an official title. Therefore, I have changed *Microbiology* to *microbiology*, *Physiology* to *physiology*, and so forth. Please also do so elsewhere.

Example: *M.D.* was changed to *MD*, and *Ph.D.* was changed to *PhD*, in keeping with Section 13.1 of the *AMA Manual of Style*.

Phrasing a query in terms of the intended readership can be well worth considering. After all, easing communication with the reader is the main goal of editing. And framing a query in terms of readers' needs can help save an editor from seeming ignorant.

Not-great wording: So, who was William Carlos Williams? [Possible reactions from author receiving query: "Are you just asking because you're interested, or should I insert an explanation? If the former, couldn't you just look it up? And should you even be editing this manuscript if you don't know who physician-poet-writer William Carlos Williams was?"]

Improved query: Perhaps consider saying who William Carlos Williams was.

Further-improved query: Will your readers know who William Carlos Williams was? If not, perhaps add a brief explanation.

In writing queries, try to avoid language that sounds accusatory, for example because it contains the word *you* in a derogatory context or says *fail*. Likewise, do not phrase requests as "Could you . . . ?" (which could reasonably elicit the response of "I could, but I won't"). Examples:

Poor query: You failed to explain what this acronym stands for. Could you define it?

Improved query: Please say what this acronym stands for. Thanks!

As noted by Deming, envisioning yourself conversing with the author can aid in formulating cordial, effective queries. For more on querying, Deming's article on this theme (Deming 2010b) is highly recommended.

Editing for Mechanics: General and Medical Aspects

Editing for mechanics includes checking items such as punctuation, grammar, spelling, capitalization, and word usage. It also can include flagging basic problems with numbers or statistics. This section will address, with a minimum of jargon, some of the most common mechanical problems to look for when editing medical manuscripts. For exhaustive information on editing for mechanics, please see such resources as *The Copyeditor's Handbook* (Einsohn and Schwartz 2019), the *AMA Manual of Style* (AMA Manual of Style Committee 2020), the exercises or quizzes accompanying both (Bűky, Schwartz, and Einsohn 2019; https://academic.oup.com/amamanualofstyle/pages/style-quizzes), and the associated answer keys.

SOME COMMON MECHANICAL ERRORS TO CORRECT

Many mechanical errors in medical manuscripts are of the same common types. Editing for mechanics entails largely being alert for and correcting these errors.

Punctuation

In medical manuscripts, the most common mechanical errors might well be those in use of *commas*. Although some aspects of comma use differ among publications and so just reflect the publication's style, most aspects do not vary. Common errors regarding the latter include lack of commas in compound sentences, omission of the comma at the end of an appositive, and omission of the comma at the end of a nonrestrictive clause.

Basically, compound sentences consist of two (or more) parts, called independent clauses, that each have both a subject and a predicate (and so are the equivalent of full sentences) and that are connected by a word, known as a coordinating conjunction, such as *and*, *but*, or *or*. Unless the parts are very short, a comma should precede the connecting word. Authors often neglect to include this comma, and thus the sentence reads like the following:

> This syndrome is incompletely understood and often ineffectively managed despite many years of research but recent advances by groups in various countries offer promise for substantial improvements in treatment within the next decade.

Properly punctuated, the sentence would be as follows:

> This syndrome is incompletely understood and often ineffectively managed despite many years of research, but recent advances by groups in various countries offer promise for substantial improvements in treatment within the next decade.

Appositives and nonrestrictive clauses add information about someone or something mentioned. Let's say the someone is "my former department head." An appositive adding information about him could be "a veterinary researcher." And a nonrestrictive clause doing so could be "who is a veterinary researcher." Thus, I could write "My former department head, a veterinary researcher, spent many years in Alaska." Or I could write "My former department head, who is a veterinary researcher, spent many years in Alaska." Either way, a comma should both precede and follow the appositive or nonrestrictive clause. Too often, authors neglect to include the second comma.

Nonrestrictive clauses add information but do not make the subject more specific. But let's say I have one department head but multiple friends, one of whom is a veterinary researcher. Then, in the latter case, "who is a veterinary researcher" makes the meaning more specific, by distinguishing this person from my other friends (for example, the one who is a musician and the one who is a swimmer). Because the clause is essential to the meaning, it would not be set off by commas. Thus, I would write "My friend who is a veterinary researcher received a grant."

Speaking of grants, here's another example of nonrestrictive and restrictive. There is only one US National Institutes of Health (NIH). Thus, the information that it funded my friend's research does not make the subject more specific and so is nonrestrictive. Accordingly, this information would be surrounded by commas; for example, I could write "The US National Institutes of Health, which funded my friend's research, has its headquarters in Maryland." However, a subject such as "the agency" is nonspecific, as there are many agencies; adding the information that it funded my friend's research narrows it down—or, in other words, is restrictive. Thus, I would write, without commas, "The agency that funded my friend's research has its headquarters in Maryland." Note that, at least in US usage, *that* generally should be used for restrictive clauses and *which* for nonrestrictive. Perhaps envision the commas surrounding nonrestrictive elements as handles with which the extra information can be lifted in and out. Ensure that the latter handle isn't missing.

By the way: The term *National Institutes of Health*, though plural in form because NIH contains multiple institutes, refers to a single entity and so takes a singular verb, such as *is*. Ditto for *Centers for Disease Control and Prevention* (CDC). Authors often omit the *s* from these names. Ensure that the *s* is present.

Often, medical manuscripts also have *semicolon* problems to correct. The most common such problem is presence of a semicolon when other punctuation, or none at all, should be used. Other than in reference lists, semicolons have only two main uses. One is to connect two closely related independent clauses. For example: "Some students like anatomy best; others prefer biochemistry." (In such instances, a period and capital letter could be substituted. Ditto for a comma and coordinating conjunction. Examples: "Some students like anatomy best. Others prefer biochemistry." and "Some students like anatomy best, but others prefer biochemistry.") The other main use is to separate lists within a list. For example: "Healthful lunch menus include grilled salmon, a baked sweet potato, and steamed broccoli; cottage cheese, fresh berries, and a low-fat muffin; and lentil curry, brown rice, and seasonal fruit." Sometimes, apparently at the prompting of misguided word-processing programs, authors follow a dependent clause with a semicolon instead of, as they should, a comma. Thus, a sentence might read, for example, "Although most patients experience no side effects of this drug; a few develop diarrhea" instead of "Although most patients experience no side effects of this drug, a few develop diarrhea." Likewise, some authors mistakenly use a semicolon, rather than a colon, to introduce a list. They may write, for example, "Clinical electives on this campus include the following; cardiology, gastroenterology, neonatology, radiation therapy, and urology" instead of "Clinical electives on this campus include the following: cardiology, gastroenterology, neonatology, radiation therapy, and urology."

Regarding *colons*: Perhaps the most common problem is their excessive use. Their main use in medical writing, other than in references, is to introduce lists. But they should be present only if the list is preceded by an introductory noun or phrase, such as "the following" or "as follows." Compare, for example, the punctuation of the sentence about healthful lunch menus and that of the (corrected) sentence about clinical electives. In the former, "include" leads directly into the list and so is not followed by a colon. In the latter, a colon indicates that "the following" introduces the list rather than being part of it.

Hyphens and dashes sometimes confuse authors—and beginning editors. A *hyphen* (-) is short. An *em dash* (—), so called because it is about the width of a letter *m*, is long. An *en dash* (–), about as wide as the letter *n*, is intermediate in length and is sometimes mistaken for a hyphen. An em dash commonly indicates a shift in thought, as in the first sentence of this paragraph. Em dashes rarely appear in scholarly medical writing, such as journal articles and grant proposals. They sometimes are used, however, in popular medical writing, such as magazine articles. Typically, spaces do not precede and follow em dashes. However, practices in this regard differ among publications. Publications also differ among themselves as to whether—and, if so, how—they use en dashes. For instance, some publications use en dashes to indicate ranges of numbers (example: 23–35), but others use hyphens for this purpose (example: 23-25). For guidance on en dashes, it is best to consult the style manual used by the target publication or the instructions provided by it; if no guidance in this regard is provided, following examples or consulting a style manual that seems appropriate makes sense.

A major use of hyphens is to connect words in a compound

modifier—that is, a group of two or more words functioning together as an adjective—that appears before a noun. Presence of the hyphen can be important to meaning; for example, "small-animal clinic" is a clinic for small animals, but a "small animal clinic" is a small clinic for animals. Hyphens should not be included, however, if the compound modifier appears later in the sentence. Thus, for example, it is proper to write "a 10-year-old boy," "a bright-red lesion," or "a high-quality project"—but "The boy was 10 years old," "The lesion was bright red," or "The project is of high quality." An exception: When the first word in a compound modifier is an adverb ending in -ly, the compound modifier should not be hyphenated even if it appears before a noun. Thus, proper punctuation would be "a rapidly expanding mass" or "a locally owned clinic" (not "a rapidly-expanding mass" or "a locally-owned clinic"). Also, a hyphen should be used if it would prevent ambiguity or misreading. For example, a recent communication stated that editors who had freelanced for a certain publisher for five years or more would have to *resign*. This statement made little sense until the context indicated that these editors would need to renew their contracts—in other words, *re-sign*. Awareness of these basic principles enables correction of many—probably most—hyphen problems in medical manuscripts.

Grammar

Often, the grammar in medical manuscripts is relatively good or easily improved. Native speakers of English commonly have an inherent sense of English grammar and make few grammatical errors. And non-native writers of medical English often have formally studied English grammar; thus, their writing tends to reflect cognizance of its rules, and any grammatical difficulties tend to be fairly easy to resolve. Also, many medical authors use grammar-checking software to help in identifying and correcting possible grammar errors. Two aspects of grammar, however, commonly pose challenges for native and non-native users of English alike. One is subject-verb agreement. The other is the evolution of grammatical norms.

Subject-verb agreement means that the number of the subject and the number of the verb should agree. For example, it is proper to write "The anatomy *course includes* dissections." or "The anatomy *courses include* dissections." Few authors would write "The anatomy *course include* dissections." or "The anatomy *courses includes* dissections." The difficulty occurs when multiple words appear between the subject and verb, such that a singular subject might incorrectly appear to be plural. Thus, for example, an author might write "The anatomy course that is available to medical students, physical therapy students, medical illustration students, medical communications students, and students in allied fields on our campuses include dissections." and not notice that "course" and "include" do not agree in number. Medical editors should be alert for such disagreement and correct it. Also, such disagreement may be a sign that a sentence is hard to follow and would benefit from restructuring or from division into more than one sentence. For example, the sentence above might read better as "Our anatomy course (which is available to medical students, physical therapy students, medical illustration students, medical communications students, and students in allied fields on our campuses) includes dissections."

Also, help ensure *parallelism*—in other words, use of the same grammatical form when two or more items appear in series. For example, "Suitable forms of exercise include jogging, rowing, and to swim" should be revised to read "Suitable forms of exercise include jogging, rowing, and swimming." And the following call for research participants—"Are you between 30 and 65 years of age and need to lose weight?"—should be recast, for instance as "Are you between 30 and 65 years of age and in need of weight loss?" or (probably better) "Are you between 30 and 65 years of age, and do you need to lose weight?"

Confusion also can reflect evolving norms regarding some grammatical constructions. For example, many authors and editors were taught not to split infinitives (for example, not to write "to rapidly increase" rather than "to increase rapidly"). Similarly, they were told not to end sentences with prepositions (for example, not to write "Such cases are appropriate to write about" rather than "Such cases are appropriate ones about which to write"). Such advice is now viewed as misguided. However, many readers still think such constructions are incorrect—and so may be distracted by them rather than focusing on the content of the writing. Therefore, such constructions often are best avoided, either by following the old norms or by rewording the material to avoid the issue (example: "Such cases are appropriate to report." or "Such cases are appropriate to publish.").

One area of recent evolution regards using *they* as a singular in instances in which a person does not identify as a *he* or a *she* or in which the sex or gender of the person is irrelevant or unspecified. Use of *they*, *them*, and *their* as singulars has long been common in informal speech ("Oh, the consultant finally got back to you? What did they say?"). However, in formal writing, such use was long deemed unsuitable. Currently, various major stylebooks, including the *AMA Manual of Style*, allow using *they* as a singular but recommend avoiding it when feasible. Alternatives can include repeating the person's name, using a noun instead of a pronoun (for example, "the respiratory therapist" rather than "they"), and using plurals (for example, rather than writing "The typical medical student worries about their student debt," writing "Typical medical students worry about their student debt.").

Spelling, Plurals, Abbreviations, and Capitalization

Spelling rarely poses major challenges in medical editing. General and medical dictionaries and spellcheckers, plus specialized such references (such as dictionaries of audiology, dentistry, or ophthalmology), usually provide the guidance needed. And with time, medical editors build their specialized vocabularies and need not consult such resources as often. An aspect that can bear attention, though, is whether to use American or British spelling, depending on the nationality of a journal. Setting your spellchecker for the requested version of English (or for the other language of the text) can help in this regard.

A common category of errors to be alert for regards irregular plurals. Many authors confuse *criterion* and *criteria*, *phenomenon* and *phenomena*, or *mitochondrion* and *mitochondria*. *Criterion*, *phenomenon*, and *mitochondrion* are singular; *criteria*, *phenomena*, and *mitochondria* are plural. Some medical and scientific terms also have irregular plurals—for example, *metastases* as the plural of *metastasis*, *vertebrae* as the plural of *vertebra*, and *genera* as the plural of *genus*. Preferred forms in such regards sometimes change over time. If in doubt, consult a suitable dictionary. And consistently use the same form. Also, remember that plurals of abbreviations consisting of all capital letters are made simply by *adding a lowercase* s (*not by adding an apostrophe and an* s). Some examples: *CBCs*, *ECGs*, and *ICUs*. Also, if you are editing material about medical or other graduates: Note that *alumnus* is the male singular, *alumna* is the female singular, *alumni* is the male plural (sometimes also used when a group includes both men and women), and *alumnae* is the female plural. Sometimes the matter can be avoided simply by referring to *a graduate* or *graduates*.

A common issue relating to plurals regards use of the word *data*. Technically, *data* is the plural of the word *datum* and so should be treated as a plural (example: "The data are . . ."). Sometimes, however, *data* functions as a mass noun similar to *information*. Some authors and editors feel strongly about whether to treat *data* as a singular or plural. For copyeditors, though, some flexibility can be advisable. If the style manual being followed or the journal's instructions to authors provide guidance on this subject, that guidance should be followed. Otherwise, reasonable approaches include choosing one convention or the other and following it consistently or using the singular or the plural depending on the context (examples: "The data shows that the latter approach is superior." but "Several data are missing from this table.").

Similar issues arise regarding *media*. This word is the plural of *medium* and so should usually be treated as a plural. For example, preferred wording generally would be "The media are a major source of health information," not "The media is a major source of health information." Similarly, a substance in which bacteria or cells are cultured in the laboratory is a *medium*, not a *media*. Hence, for example: "We replaced the medium daily." but "We compared the growth rates in the following media."

A few words on *abbreviations*, including *acronyms* (abbreviations formed from the first letters of some or all words in a phrase): In some styles, including AMA, abbreviations normally do not contain periods. Thus, proper style would be to write "Dr Doe, of the AMA, and Col Poe, of the USPHS, discussed CDC and NIH findings about MIs, STIs, and UTIs in HMOs." (Note: Although it embodies proper abbreviation style, this sentence is dreadful. Not only does it make little sense, but placing so many abbreviations so close together hampers readability.)

Typically, terms should be written out in full on first appearance, with the abbreviation following in parentheses. For example, standard practice would be to write "adenosine triphosphate (ATP)" and thereafter just to write "ATP." (In AP style, though, the term is used in full on first mention, without the abbreviation in parentheses. Thereafter the abbreviation is used, with the assumption that readers can infer from the context what it stands for.) If an entity is better known by its abbreviation than by its full name, a case can be made for presenting the abbreviation first and then its full name in parentheses; for example, one might justifiably say "HIPAA (the Health Insurance Portability and Accountability Act) requires that . . . ." (Please note: The proper abbreviation is *HIPAA*—not *HIPPA*, as authors sometimes write.) If a document is long and audience members might not read the parts in order or might not read the document at a single session, defining abbreviations the first time they appear in a given section can serve readers well. Likewise, including a table or list of abbreviations and their definitions can help; indeed, some journals require doing so.

In some styles, some common abbreviations can be used without definition. For example, AMA style allows use, without such expansion, of *AIDS*, *CME*, *COVID-19*, *DNA*, *HIV*, and *URL*, among others. Likewise, some specialized journals allow undefined use of some abbreviations that readers in their fields invariably know.

Usually, an abbreviation should be used only if a term will be used at least a few times; otherwise, the space saved is not worth the possible confusion. Also, authors should use mainly well-established abbreviations. They should coin few, if any, abbreviations of their own.

Because the same acronym can have different meanings in different fields, acronyms can especially confuse in multidisciplinary contexts. Even when GC is explicitly defined as "general counsel" or PID is explicitly defined as "persistent identifier," a physician may struggle to avoid thinking "gonococcus" and "pelvic inflammatory disease." And used in the title of an article, does AI refer to artificial intelligence or artificial insemination?

Medical editors should be alert for common problems in abbreviation use. These problems include failure to define abbreviations when needed, use of nonstandard abbreviations, and excessive abbreviation use. Particular stringency is warranted in editing presentations; whereas article readers who forget what an abbreviation stands for can look back for the definition, listeners to a presentation cannot do so and therefore may become lost.

Two abbreviations deserving attention are *e.g.* (which stands for the Latin *exempli gratia*, meaning "for example") and *i.e.* (which stands for the Latin *id est*, meaning "that is"). Authors often confuse the two or think they are synonyms. Similarly, readers often confuse them. In editing manuscripts, check whether these abbreviations have been used correctly. And to prevent confusion, consider replacing them with "for example" and "that is." The increase in clarity can be well worth the slight increase in length.

In medical writing, the most common problem regarding *capitalization* appears to be its excessive use. Many authors capitalize too many words. For example, they mistakenly capitalize the names of scientific disciplines, medical specialties, and diseases. Terms such as *biochemistry* and *internal medicine* should be capitalized only when appearing within official titles (for example, *Department of Biochemistry and Biophysics* or the journal *Annals of Internal Medicine*). Similarly, terms such as *amyotrophic lateral sclerosis, diabetes mellitus,* and *rheumatoid arthritis* should not be capitalized in normal text, although the corresponding abbreviations (such as ALS, DM, and RA) consist of all capitals. Also, in disease names containing the name of the person, only the person's name should be capitalized; hence *Alzheimer disease* (not *Alzheimer Disease*).

When a genus and species are stated, the former but not the latter should be capitalized. Hence: *Staphylococcus aureus, Felis catus,* and *Homo sapiens.* Please note that the genus and species names should be italicized.

MEDICAL WORD USAGE

Copyediting also includes checking for proper usage of terms. Medical and general dictionaries can aid in this regard. In addition, medical editors should be alert for common problems in medical usage. This section discusses some of these problems.

Commonly Confused Terms

Some terms common in medical writing also are commonly confused. Here are some to be especially alert for. The usage chapter in the *AMA Manual of Style* discusses many more.

Die from/Die of: The correct wording is *die of* (not *died from*). For example, "The patient died of heart failure."

Incidence/Prevalence: Incidence refers to the number or rate of new cases of a condition. *Prevalence* refers to how common the condition is. For example, if last year 123 out of 100,000 people in a given population developed the mythical condition "editors' disease," the incidence of editors' disease in that population last year would be 123 per 100,000 people. But if according to a survey last week, 45 per 100,000 people in that population currently had editors' disease, the prevalence of editors' disease in that population at that time would be 45 per 100,000 people. One way to remember the difference between *incidence* and *prevalence* is to think of the terms *incident* and *prevail.*

Patient/Case: A patient is a person receiving medical care. A case is an instance. Thus, one would write "We examined 10 patients with this syndrome" but "We analyzed 10 cases of this syndrome" or "We reported

10 cases of this syndrome." Technically, someone with a disease is a patient only if receiving medical care. Thus, in other contexts, they should not be referred to as patients. Rather, they could be referred to as people with the disease or, if they are enrolled in a study, research participants with the disease.

Preventative/Preventive: These terms are synonyms. The latter, being shorter, is preferred.

Sensitivity/Specificity: Sensitivity regards how good a test is at detecting a condition. *Specificity* regards whether it detects only instances of a condition. For example, a test that always detects a given disease if present—in other words, that has no false negatives—is highly sensitive. And a test that never indicates that the disease is present when in fact it is absent—in other words, that has no false positives—is highly specific. Ideally, tests are both sensitive and specific.

Signs/Symptoms: In everyday language, these terms tend to be used interchangeably. In medicine, however, they have distinct meanings. *Signs* are manifestations of disease that are observable by others—for example, fever, swelling, or a rash. *Symptoms* are observable only to the person experiencing them; examples include pain, nausea, and itching.

Use/Utilize: In an effort to sound scholarly, authors often say *utilize* rather than *use*. However, the former, simpler term almost always is preferable. Also, *utilize* tends to indicate using an item for other than its original purpose. (Example: "When performing the home assay, he utilized a napkin ring to keep the tube upright.")

As medical editors, we also should use (not utilize!) terms in our own field properly. I recently encountered a sentence that read "He spends most of his day writing and editing grants and studies." Such a statement might be fine in informal speech. However, a grant is funding received (for example, to do research)—not the request for the funding. And a study is a piece of research, not the report of the research. More exact ways to word the sentence include the following: "He spends most of his day writing and editing grant proposals and scientific papers." and "He spends most of his day writing and editing grant applications and journal articles."

Nomenclature

Some areas of medicine have standardized systems of terminology—in other words, standard nomenclature. For example, there are standard ways to designate blood groups, cancer stages, heart murmurs, genes, and mental disorders. Especially when editing relatively technical materials such as journal articles and grant proposals, medical editors should be aware of such nomenclature and know how to check it. The *AMA Manual of Style* provides extensive guidance on nomenclature in various medical fields; for example, in the print version of the 11th edition (AMA Manual of Style Committee 2020), the chapter on nomenclature runs nearly 300 pages; as well as specifying nomenclature to use, it lists references for further information. *The CSE Manual: Scientific Style and Format for Authors, Editors, and Publishers* (Council of Science Editors Style Manual Task Force 2024) also includes guidance in such regards.

Generic Versus Brand Names

Medical writing often contains drug names, and a medical editor's tasks include checking the use of these names. Normally, the generic name (for example, *ibuprofen*) should be used, not the brand name (for example, *Advil* or *Motrin*). Exceptions exist, however. One exception is when the brand is relevant—for instance, when the writing regards an aspect of a particular brand of a drug. Another is when the readership knows a drug mainly by its brand name. In these instances, both the brand name and the generic name should be included. As shown earlier in this paragraph, brand names but not generic names should be capitalized. An example of proper capitalization: "In general, you should write *diazepam* rather than *Valium*, *furosemide* rather than *Lasix*, and *rosuvastatin* rather than *Crestor*."

Eponyms and Toponyms

Many diseases, medical procedures, and the like are named after people. Thus, for example, authors may write of Alzheimer disease, the Babinski sign, the Billroth II operation, DeBakey forceps, Down syndrome, the tetralogy of Fallot, Trendelenburg position, and the Valsalva maneuver. Medical editors should keep several items in mind when working with such name-containing terms, or *eponyms*. First, in both AMA style and CSE style (and thus most medical journals), current practice is not to use the possessive form of the person's name; thus, for example, the preferred form is *Crohn disease* (not *Crohn's disease*). (In some other styles, such as AP and APA, whether to use the possessive varies among terms.) Second, in the eponym, the person's name is capitalized, but the other word or words are not. Third, remember that eponyms can be confusing, both because they do not describe what they refer to and because some eponyms are used only in some countries. Therefore, it can be wise to add or substitute a more descriptive term (for example, *chronic adrenocortical insufficiency* for *Addison disease*). Finally, adjectives derived from eponyms should not be capitalized. Hence, for example, a manuscript should say *parkinsonian* (not *Parkinsonian*) *tremor.*

Some medical terms incorporate names of places and so are called *toponyms.* Examples include *Lyme disease* (named after Lyme, Connecticut), *Coxsackievirus* (after Coxsackie, New York), and *Rift Valley fever* (after the Rift Valley in Kenya). Capitalization conventions for eponyms also apply to toponyms. Recent practice has been to avoid naming diseases and their causative agents after places, as doing so can be stigmatizing. For example, the "World Health Organization Best Practices for the Naming of New Human Infectious Diseases" (World Health Organization 2015) advises that names for newly discovered diseases contain descriptive terms rather than names of people, places, types of animals, or cultural or occupational groups.

UNBIASED, RESPECTFUL WORDING

Medical writing often regards patients, health professionals, medical scientists, or other people. Thus, medical copyediting includes helping to ensure that people are referred to in ways that are unbiased and otherwise respectful and that honor their preferences. Doing so can pose challenges—in part because guidelines keep evolving and in part because even members of the same group can differ in preferences. However, knowledge of key norms and common issues can aid considerably, as can awareness of pertinent resources. Helpful resources include the section "Inclusive Language" in the *AMA Manual of Style* (AMA Manual of Style Committee 2020), online updates to this manual (https://academic.oup.com/amamanualofstyle/pages/about/updates-to-the-manual), "Inclusive Language" in *The CSE Manual* (Council of Science Editors Style Manual Task Force 2024), "Bias-Free Language Guidelines" in the *Publication Manual of the American Psychological Association* (American Psychological Association 2020), and "Inclusive Language and Minimizing Bias" in *The Chicago Manual of Style* (University of Chicago Press Editorial Staff 2024). Also useful are *The Conscious Style Guide* (Yin 2024), the "disabilities" entry and other relevant entries (such as that on "gender, sex and sexual orientation") in *The Associated Press Stylebook* (Associated Press

2024), and the *Disability Language Style Guide* (National Center on Disability and Journalism 2021) from the National Center on Disability and Journalism.

Copyediting includes ensuring that wording is inclusive. Some examples of revising for inclusivity are as follows:

Original: A surgical resident must work long hours. Therefore he has little time for other pursuits. (as if all surgical residents were male)
Revised: Surgical residents must work long hours. Therefore they have little time for other pursuits. *or* Surgical residents, who must work long hours, have little time for other pursuits.

Original: Although this condition is most common in gay men, it also occurs in the general population. (as if gay men were not part of the general population)
Revised: Although this condition is most common in gay men, it also occurs in other people.

Original: This service is available to adults and seniors. (as if older adults were not still adults)
Revised: The service is available to adults of all ages. *or* This service is available to adults.

Also consider details that may contribute to stereotypes. For example, in editing a series of feature articles about clinicians or researchers, seek consistency between genders as to whether information about family status is included.

Race and ethnicity also require copyeditorial attention. Sometimes that attention consists of recommending that their mention be deleted; for example, only if relevant should a patient's or other person's race or ethnicity be noted. If race or ethnicity is mentioned—for example, in a report of a case where this aspect is pertinent, or in the demographic data on a population studied—appropriate terminology should be used. For example, current guidelines such as those in the *AMA Manual of Style* and *The CSE Manual* call for using the terms *Black* and *White* and for capitalizing them.

Copyeditors also should consider wording regarding age. Terms such as *senior citizens* and *the elderly* may have unwanted connotations. And although *older adults* is comfortably neutral, it can be overly vague. (Does it mean people over 50 years of age? over 65? over 80?) In general, best practice is to specify the age range of the group being discussed. Also check for such specificity in writing about children. And especially in technical medical writing such as journal articles, make sure that terms regarding age are used exactly. According to the *AMA Manual of Style* (AMA Manual of Style Committee 2020, Section 11.7), respective age ranges are *neonates* or *newborns*, birth to 1 month of age; *infants*, 1 month to 1 year; *children* (including *boys* and *girls*), 1 to 12 years, or sometimes birth to 12 years; *adolescents*, 13 to 17 years; and *adults*, 18 years and above.

In general, a female adult should be referred to as a *woman* and a male adult as a *man*; using the terms *female* and *male* as nouns to refer to individuals tends to be dehumanizing. Thus, for example, "The patient was a 57-year-old female." should be edited to read "The patient was a 57-year-old woman." The nouns *female* and *male* may, however, be used, generally in the plural, when referring to groups containing both children and adults. (Example: "One restroom was for females and the other for males.") And *male* and *female* as nouns may be used to refer to animals. (Example: "Of the mice exhibiting this behavior, 17 were males and 14 were females.")

Much medical writing is about people with diseases, disabilities, or other conditions. Wording in this regard merits copyeditorial checking. Melodramatic, sometimes demeaning wording such as "victim" or "suffers" generally should be replaced. Examples of appropriate edits include changing "cancer victim" to "woman with cancer" or "man with cancer," and changing "suffers from asthma" to "has asthma." Typically, the favored wording is "person first"—for example, "people with diabetes" rather than "diabetics," and "people with schizophrenia" rather than "schizophrenics"—so as to show that the medical condition does not define the person's identity. Some people, however, do consider their medical condition an integral part of their identity and so prefer that it come first (for example, "deaf scientist" or "autistic person"). When writing about groups of people with given medical conditions, organizations focusing on those conditions can provide guidance on preferred terminology, as can resources listed earlier in this section. When editing a piece about an individual with a given condition, it can be worth checking the person's preference.

Wording about assistive technologies also bears checking. In everyday speech, people sometimes say "confined to a wheelchair." However, the neutral "uses a wheelchair" is preferable—especially as a wheelchair tends to liberate rather than confine a person whose mobility would otherwise be more limited. Consider how you would edit this passage: "The patient suffered from Alzheimer's disease. She was wheelchair bound."

If an editor's duties extend to visuals, the visuals also should be considered regarding inclusivity and avoidance of bias. For example, if an image portrays a group of health professionals, are sufficiently diverse individuals shown in various roles? Do images of patients avoid perpetuating stereotypes? If not, what might be done?

A final issue, also discussed earlier in this chapter, regards choice of pronouns. Until recently, style manuals generally said to avoid using *they* as a singular pronoun. However, use of *they* as a singular pronoun is now deemed acceptable in at least two instances. One instance is when an individual, such as someone identifying as neither male nor female, prefers being referred to as *they* rather than *he* or *she*. The other instance is when the gender of a person is unknown or irrelevant (Example: "The chief administrative officer of the unit should review each application with regard to criteria A, B, D, and F. They also should certify that matching funds will be available."). However, the latter use can distract from the content, as some readers remain under the impression that *they* should not be used as a singular. Therefore, where feasible, a copyeditor may find it preferable to pursue an alternative, such as repeating the noun (rather than using a pronoun) or making the noun plural.

NUMBERS AND STATISTICS

Medical writing commonly includes many numbers. Medical copyeditors check whether these numbers are in the proper format. To some extent, they also check whether the numbers seem to make sense.

Editors from the humanities may be accustomed to spelling out numbers 0 through 100 in words. Those from social science or journalism may be accustomed to doing so for numbers less than 10. In technical medical writing, such as that following AMA or CSE style, numerals are used even for small numbers. For example, one would write of 5 patients, 3 groups, or 7 investigators. An exception is that even in the latter styles, a numeral generally should not appear at the beginning of a sentence. Thus, the practice would be to write "We treated 5 patients" but "Five patients were treated." To avoid writing out a long number at the beginning of a sentence, an editor can rearrange the sentence or precede the number with a word or brief phrase. For instance, rather than revising

"748 samples were analyzed" to read "Seven hundred forty-eight samples were analyzed," consider revising it to read (depending on the context) "We analyzed 748 samples," "In total, 748 samples were analyzed," or "Then 748 samples were analyzed."

A specialized point of AMA style is the use of a *thin space* to separate groups of digits. In the United States, commas commonly are used to separate groups of three digits in large numbers (example: 2,272,561,025). In some other countries, periods serve this purpose (example: 2.272.561.025). By using thin spaces (example: 2 272 561 025), AMA style avoids the need to decide between these conventions. To make a thin space in Microsoft Word, you can go to the symbols menu and specify insertion of Unicode character 2009.

Authors often present percentages to excessive numbers of decimal places. For example, if 17 out of 41 patients had a given finding, they may write that 41.4634% of patients did so. However, such a number conveys a false sense of exactness. Normally, if the denominator (for example, the total number of patients) is 100 or less, the percentage should be presented as a whole number. And otherwise, one decimal place usually suffices. Also, be sure that the writing includes the raw numbers, not only the percentages. Does the 33% represent 1 of the 3 patients studied (in which case the numbers probably are too low for percentages to be meaningful) or 330 of the 1000 patients studied? Does a 90% decrease in death rate mean a decrease from 10% to 1% or a decrease from 10 in a million to 1 in a million? The implications can be very different.

One year in my medical editing course, a student pleaded, "Please don't tell me I need to check the math." Normally, medical copyeditors need not check higher math; if journal articles contain differential equations or sophisticated mathematical models, it is up to the authors and peer reviewers (and sometimes a statistical editor or specialized content editor) to check their validity. However, medical copyeditors *are* expected to be numerate and to be alert for arithmetic errors, mathematical inconsistencies, and the like. Do the percentages of a group add up to 89 instead of 100? Is something that decreased by half reported as having declined 200%? Does a number in a table differ from the corresponding number in the text? Does the text say *decrease* but a graph show an increase? Is a patient's blood pressure listed as 520/85 mm Hg? In such circumstances, the copyeditor should query the author to resolve the discrepancy.

And what about statistics? Medical copyeditors are not expected to be statisticians. However, some acquaintance with statistics (for example, from a biostatistics course) can aid in medical copyediting and especially in substantive editing. Even without such background, medical editors can be alert for some basic problems. One problem regards *P* values (which, in essence, represent the likelihood that a finding is a fluke rather than indicating a true difference between groups). By definition, a *P* value cannot exceed 1, as the likelihood of something occurring cannot exceed 100%. Accordingly, if a reported *P* value is more than 1, the author should be queried. A low *P value* (for example, .001) indicates a low probability that the finding was a fluke and thus a high likelihood that there truly was a difference. And by convention, .05 commonly is used as the cutoff point for statistical significance; in other words, if chances appear less than 1 in 20 that a finding was a fluke, the thought is that the finding probably was real. However, this cutoff point is not magic, and sometimes researchers may, for example, choose a more stringent cutoff point. Also, statistical significance does not always mean clinical significance. For example, a difference may be real but so small that it would not make any difference in patient care. Such items may be helpful to keep in mind in copyediting.

Normally, if a number is less than 1, a zero precedes the decimal point, to make clear that the number is a decimal. For example, writing 0.325 helps prevent misreading .325 as 325 (which could cause major problems if, for example, the number regards a recommended drug dose). AMA style, however, contains an exception: As shown in the previous paragraph, *P* values appear without the leading zero. The reason is that *P* values, being probabilities, cannot exceed 1 and therefore do not risk being misread in this regard. Some other styles, however, such as Council of Science Editors (CSE) style, include the leading zero in *P* values. Copyeditors should follow the journal's instructions or the specified style manual in determining whether to include a leading zero when reporting *P* values.

Another item to be alert for: Many medical journal articles include *confidence intervals*, which are analogous to margins of error. For example, if an estimated value is 5.3 and statistical calculations indicate that, with 95% certainty, the actual value lies between 4.3 and 6.3, the 95% confidence interval would be from 4.3 to 6.3. The estimated value must lie within the confidence interval. If it does not, the author should be queried to resolve the discrepancy.

More advanced copyediting, and especially substantive editing, may include additional checking to help ensure that the presented statistics are both plausible and presented in keeping with appropriate conventions.

Extensive guidance in the latter regard appears in *How to Report Statistics in Medicine: Annotated Guidelines for Authors, Editors, and Reviewers*, 2nd edition, by Thomas A. Lang and Michelle Secic (Lang and Secic 2006). Stylebooks such as the *AMA Manual of Style* (AMA Manual of Style Committee 2020) also provide considerable guidance on statistics and their presentation. Editors without a background in statistics may find it useful to obtain such background.

YES, SYNTAX TOO

Syntax—in other words, the arrangement of words or phrases in a sentence—also merits the copyeditor's attention. When syntax is so poor that the sentence is ambiguous, inaccurate, or preposterous, the copyeditor should remedy the syntax. If uncertain whether the revised wording conveys the intended meaning, the copyeditor should query the author.

Some humorous examples, adapted from work I have encountered:

- While in college, my cat developed kidney disease.
  (*Possible revision*: While I was in college, my cat developed kidney disease.)

- She was residing in her mother's house, who was suffering from arthritis.
  (*Possible revision*: She was residing at the house of her mother, who had arthritis.)

- It is necessary to increase awareness of disease spread among farmers, veterinary workers, and consumers.
  (Here it sounds as if the disease is spreading among these population groups. A potential revision of this sentence is "It is necessary to increase farmers', veterinary workers', and consumers' awareness of disease spread.")

More seriously, the following four categories of poor syntax often occur and should be cured. The first category consists of dangling participles and related dislocations in which what a part of the sentence grammatically modifies is not what the part of the sentence really refers to. Some examples:

- Once sedated, we cleaned the wound.

  (Presumably, the patient—not the care team—was sedated. Suggested rewrite: "Once the patient was sedated, we cleaned the wound.")

- After sampling the blood, the pigs will be euthanized.

  (Taken literally, this sentence indicates that the pigs sample the blood. Although having laboratory animals help with research could be convenient, it seems unlikely that the pigs did so. Possible revisions of this sentence include "After the blood is sampled, the pigs will be euthanized" and "After sampling the blood, we will euthanize the pigs.")

- After closing the abdomen, the right jugular vein was catheterized.

  (Hmmm, it could be helpful to have veins assist with surgery.)

- Walking down the hall, my heart was pounding.

  (So, hearts can walk.)

- After purifying the material, the samples were analyzed.

  (Well, you get the idea.)

The second category consists of misplacement of the word *only*. The word *only* should be adjacent to what it modifies. Yet authors often put it elsewhere in the sentence. For example, referring to veterinarians specializing in feline medicine, someone might write "These specialists only treat cats." Taken literally, this wording means that these veterinarians just treat cats; they don't feed them, house them, play with them, groom them, sell them, or whatever. To convey exactly what was meant, the authors should write "These specialists treat only cats" or perhaps "These specialists treat cats only."

The third category to be mentioned regards antecedents of pronouns such as *it*, *he*, *she*, and *they*. Sometimes writing is structured such that readers cannot readily discern what the pronoun refers to—or is structured such that the pronoun seems to refer to the wrong thing. An example of the latter:

- Only the researcher and the researcher's advisor will have access to the transcripts. They will be destroyed after the minimum three-year post-research requirement.

(Note: As the researcher's advisor, I didn't especially want to be destroyed after three years. Therefore, I suggested changing "They" to "The transcripts.")

A related problem is the use of the word *this* without a noun after it. In this situation, it can be unclear whether the *this* refers to, for example, the entire concept expressed in the previous sentence or a specific noun in that sentence. The solution usually is to provide, or suggest, a noun immediately after the *this* to make clear what is being referred to.

A fourth category is *stacked nouns*—that is, use of a series of consecutive nouns, such that the relationship among the nouns is unclear or that the reader must pause to infer the relationship. A nontechnical example is "student luncheon speaker"; is the person a luncheon speaker who is a student or a speaker at a student luncheon? Stacked nouns can be especially confusing if preceded by an adjective, as in "excellent staff promotion committee meeting schedule"; does the *excellent* refer to *staff*, *schedule*, or something else? Perhaps consider how you would revise the following, taken from recently edited manuscripts: "Texas panhandle region cattle," "physically able workforce reduction," "inflammatory cascade and uterine contraction associated genes," and "naturally transient gene expression data."

A final problem related somewhat to syntax is use of mixed metaphors—in other words, conflicting metaphors in the same sentence or passage. For example, I encountered the sentence "This milestone opened the door to a tidal wave of. . . ." Conjures some interesting images.

Editing for Conformity with a Publication's Style

Copyediting, including medical copyediting, also entails ensuring compliance with the publication's style. But what does *style* mean in this context? How can a copyeditor keep track of it? The following sections address these questions.

STYLE IN THE MEDICAL EDITING SENSE

Some aspects of English are invariably, or almost invariably, either right or wrong. The word *the* is spelled *t-h-e*, not *x-y-z*. A simple declarative sentence ends with a period, not an ampersand. The past tense of *draw* is *drew*, not *drawed*. However, preferences in some other regards vary from style manual to style manual, from journal to journal, or otherwise from venue to venue. These preferences constitute a publication's *style*. In this sense, style does not mean a characteristic personal manner of expression—as in the styles of Faulkner, Fitzgerald, and Hemingway (or, in the medical literary realm, the styles of Klass, Ofri, and Verghese). Rather, it designates a set of conventions followed.

Earlier parts of this chapter referred to such differences in style. For example, it was noted that different publications follow different conventions regarding which numbers to write in words and which numbers to present as numerals. The following are some other aspects of style that medical editors may need to be alert for.

Serial comma: In the United States, scholarly writing styles, including AMA style, include use of the serial comma—for example, the comma before the *and* in "anatomy, biochemistry, and physiology." However, AP style, commonly used in newspapers and news releases, does not routinely include the serial comma; thus, the corresponding list would read "anatomy, biochemistry and physiology."

Placement of quotation marks relative to other punctuation: In the usual US style, the closing quotation mark follows the comma or period, regardless of whether the comma or period is part of the quoted material. Thus, for example, the style would be to write the following: This morning I read Atul Gawande's essay "Education of a Knife," and this afternoon I read his essay "When Doctors Make Mistakes." In the usual British style, however, the comma or period appears before the closing quotation mark only if part of the quoted material. Hence, for example: This morning I read Atul Gawande's essay 'The Education of a Knife', and this afternoon I read his essay 'When Doctors Make Mistakes'. Also, as shown in these examples, usual US style is to use double quotation marks (and to reserve single quotation marks for quotes within quotes); usual British style is the reverse.

Preferred spellings: Other style differences between US and British English regard preferred spellings of some words. US style would be to write "tumors harboring" and "The pediatrician analyzed the color of the feces." The corresponding items in British style would be "tumours harbouring" and "The paediatrician analysed the colour of the faeces." Setting your spellchecker in Word accordingly can help ensure that the English is in the appropriate country's style. Even within the same country, preferred spellings can differ among publications or institutions. Also, words evolve over time; thus, in multiple styles, *e-mail* has become *email*, *Internet* has become *internet*, *Web site* has become *website*, and *under way* has become *underway*.

Number style: As noted earlier, even numbers less than 10 generally appear as numerals in technical medical publications. However, medical writing for general readerships tends not to follow this convention. Also, as mentioned, style for formatting numbers—for example, use of commas versus use of thin spaces—can differ among publications.

Citation style: Publications differ among themselves in the style used for citing references in text. Some journals cite sources by name and date—for example, "Recent research indicates that taste perception is more complex than previously believed (Egan 2024)." In this style, references then appear in a list alphabetized by author. Other journals use numbers to cite references—for example, "Recent research indicates that taste perception is more complex than previously believed.[3]" The latter style can be associated either with a numbered alphabetized reference list or with a list in which references are numbered in the order in which they appear in the text. Within these two main types of citation style, variations also exist—for instance, regarding how the name and date are punctuated, whether the number appears as a superscript or in parentheses, and where the number appears relative to punctuation.

Reference style: Despite attempts over the years to standardize reference styles, medical journals differ among themselves in reference format in reference lists. For example, in APA style, in which articles are cited by author and date, the reference for the article cited above would be

Egan, J. M. (2024). Physiological integration of taste and metabolism. *New England Journal of Medicine*, 390(18), 1699–1710. https://doi.org/10.1056/NEJMra2304578

In AMA style, a style in which articles are cited by number, the corresponding reference would be

3. Egan JM. Physiological integration of taste and metabolism. *N Engl J Med.* 2024;390(18):1699-1710. doi: 10.1056/NEJMra2304578

Likewise, medical books differ among themselves in reference style. Authors' and editors' use of reference management software allows automatic formatting of citations and references in the requested style. However, checking still is needed, as such software and its input are imperfect. Among items to check are the following:

- whether all author names are in the proper format
- whether all article titles follow the requested style (either "up style," with all major words capitalized, or "down style," with only the first word and proper nouns capitalized)
- whether the requested style is consistently followed for whether journal titles are abbreviated or written out in full
- whether all other required elements (such as volume and year) are included
- whether every reference complies with any requested convention regarding the use of italics and boldface
- whether all punctuation and spacing are as required

Also, if the references are to include *DOIs* (digital object identifiers, which are codes that provide persistent online access), copyediting includes checking for their presence.

A CRUCIAL TOOL: STYLE SHEETS

So, how can you keep track of all the style requirements and style choices, and thus help ensure that the style in a manuscript is both correct and consistent? The answer is a *style sheet*—one or more pages specifying aspects of style for a given project. Sometimes an editorial supervisor provides a standard style sheet for an institution or periodical; the copyeditor then adds information specific to the project. Other times, the copyeditor alone prepares the style sheet. Some items on the style sheet can, and should, be specified before the editing begins. Others are added as the editing progresses and items must be looked up or decided.

To take an example: Imagine that you are editing a paper that will be submitted to a medical journal. At the top of your style sheet, you might write the manuscript's title, the authors' names, the name and contact information of the author you will communicate with, and the journal where the paper will be submitted, along with a link to the journal's instructions to authors. You will then see what, if anything, the instructions to authors say about style and format. You will also notice whether the instructions specify a style manual to follow; if they do, you would note it on your style sheet. If no style manual is specified, you might note which one seems most suited to use as fallback. You would then start developing your style sheet. Based on the journal instructions, the style manual (if any), and your own knowledge of norms in the field, you could list on your style sheet such items as whether the serial comma will be used, which conventions will be followed for numbers, how subheadings should be formatted, how references are to be cited in the text, and what reference format is to be used in the reference list. The style sheet also should include an alphabetized list of words, phrases, and abbreviations that you check and so now can easily recheck. Examples (for instance, of properly formatted references) can be helpful to include. The style sheet will evolve as the editing progresses. For example, you may find that the manuscript includes dates; after checking what format the journal uses or the style manual specifies for dates, you would indicate this information on the style sheet.

So, what can a style sheet look like? The appearance can differ somewhat, depending on the nature of the project, the preferences of the editor, and preferences of others. What's important is not that the style sheet itself appear in a "right" format but rather that it help ensure that the document being edited conforms to the requested style and is mechanically sound. Appendix 1 contains a fictional example of a style sheet for a journal article and demonstrates its use in editing the abstract of the article; Appendix 2 shows a style sheet suitable for editing a medically related article for a general readership. In addition, an example of an extensive style sheet appears in *The Copyeditor's Handbook* (Einsohn and Schwartz 2019, 60–63). Shorter sample style sheets appear in answer keys to some exercises in *The Copyeditor's Workbook* (Bűky, Schwartz, and Einsohn 2019, 238–39, 244, 278–79, 284–85, 334, 348, 357–58).

A style sheet can help ensure that your editing remains consistent, even if you return to an editing project weeks or months later. It can help ensure consistency among projects. If more than one editor will work on a publication, it can help ensure consistency among them. It also can help ensure consistency among members of a team, such as editorial supervisors, copyeditors, and proofreaders. Although style sheets are not routinely shared with authors, sharing them with authors who are especially attuned to editing can aid communication.

Editing Tables and Figures for Mechanics and Style

Medical copyediting also can include editing tables and figures for journal articles and other communications. Like text, tables and figures can be edited both in general and to meet style requirements of a given venue.

This section will touch on aspects to consider. Sources of more detailed guidance include relevant sections of style manuals, the applicable style quizzes from the *AMA Style* manual website, the chapter "Tables, Graphs, and Art" in *The Copyeditor's Handbook* (Einsohn and Schwartz 2019), the American Medical Writers Association Essential Skills Workbook on tables and graphs (Hamilton 2012), and journals' instructions to authors. Also of help are the *Clinical Chemistry* articles "Put Your Best Figure Forward: Line Graphs and Scattergrams" (Annesley 2010a), "Bars and Pies Make Better Desserts Than Figures" (Annesley 2010b), and "Bring Your Best to the Table" (Annesley 2010c). As well as providing guidance, these openly accessible articles contain exercises on correcting problems in graphs or tables.

Regardless of whether you are working with a table or a figure, check several basic items.

- In a document such as a journal article or grant proposal, make sure that every table and every figure is mentioned in the text (and that every mentioned table or figure is indeed provided). Also, make sure that the mention is near the beginning of the relevant content's discussion, so readers know to look at the table or figure promptly; a common problem is to refer to the table or figure too late.
- Make sure each table or figure has a clear and accurate title or caption.
- Check that the content of the table or figure and that of the text are consistent. Query about any discrepancies.
- Likewise, look for consistency among figures or tables. For example, if groups are listed in a given order in the first of a series of tables, they should appear in the same order in the other tables in the series. Likewise, if circles represent the experimental group and triangles the control group in one graph, the reverse should not be done in another graph.
- Make sure that each table or figure is understandable on its own, without reading the main document text. For example, in a table or figure, the study groups should not be designated merely as Group A and Group B; rather, descriptive terms (for example, "Vitamin D Group" and "Placebo Group") should be used.
- Ensure that the tables and figures are being provided in the way requested. For example, some journals want tables and figures to

be embedded at relevant places in the text, others want them all to appear at the end of the manuscript, and others want to receive them as separate files.

In tables, additional items deserve checking. A basic such item is whether a table even is needed. In general, if all the content from a table can be stated in a single reasonable-length sentence, a table probably is unnecessary. Also check whether abbreviations in the table (other than, for example, those for standard units of measure) are defined. And check whether the definitions are provided in the way required. (For example, in some journals, abbreviation-defining and other footnotes in tables are designated by superscript lowercase letters, because superscript numbers might sometimes be mistaken for exponents.) Check whether elements in the table are properly aligned, in keeping with the instructions provided or the style manual being used. Also be on the lookout for items that seem implausible and therefore should be queried about. (Was the median age of women in the study really 505 years, or perhaps should it have been 50.5 years?) And be alert for numbers that do not seem to add up, averages that seem inconsistent with the data, and the like. Of course, also do basic copyediting, such as checking spelling and grammar.

For figures, such as diagrams and graphs, copyediting includes at least editing the accompanying text, such as legends or captions. Of course, this text should be mechanically sound, without errors in grammar, spelling, punctuation, or usage. It also should be consistent with the content of the figure and should be understandable without reading the main article text. Also, the copyediting can include ensuring that items such as figure legends are submitted in the way requested. For example, some journals want figure legends to be presented as a separate list, rather than appearing below the figures as in the published article. Similarly, copyediting before submission may include helping ensure that figures are in the requested electronic format. If figures are being reproduced from elsewhere, the copyeditor may need to ascertain whether the required permissions, if any, have been obtained and to check whether appropriate credit lines are present. Likewise, if a photograph includes a patient or other person, the copyeditor's duties may include ensuring that either the person is unrecognizable (for example, because only a small square of skin is shown) or that written permission to publish the photograph has been obtained from the person (or from the parent, guardian, or other appropriate individual). Long gone are the days when simply printing a dark rectangle over a person's eyes was considered sufficient to maintain anonymity.

Rarely does copyediting include making major changes in a figure. However, it may include recommending whether to retain a figure—such as one that enlivened a talk on the research but can be omitted or replaced by a sentence in the corresponding journal article. Copyediting also may include ensuring that the axes and data points in a graph or the structures in a diagram are clearly labeled. Sometimes it includes suggesting technical improvements in a figure—for example, recommending that the author adjust the contrast in a photo, crop a photo to include only the portion of interest, make the main lines in a graph thicker than the axes so viewers will focus on the content, use other colors in a figure so viewers with color perception difficulties ("colorblindness") can better distinguish the elements, or add a scale bar to a photomicrograph. In some circumstances, manuscript editors may suggest deeper changes—such as redesigning a flowchart to make it less convoluted, ensuring that the baseline of a graph is zero to help avoid misinterpretation, using a different type of graph in order to represent content more clearly, or combining two or more figures into a composite. Such suggestions, however, tend to move beyond copyediting to *substantive editing*—the topic of the next chapter.

Beyond Copyediting Per Se

A copyeditor's work sometimes extends beyond copyediting in the narrow sense. In some contexts, it includes preparing *alt text* so people who use screen readers because of print disabilities can discern the content of images. It can include *tagging* manuscripts—for instance, inserting codes to indicate levels of headings—to guide document design. Especially at magazines, it can include *fact-checking* to ensure that every bit of information is correct and that the overall piece is on target (Borel 2023). Online resources, colleagues, and more can aid in learning these skills. Knowing the basics of medical copyediting provides a sound foundation.

Key Points

- Copyediting helps ensure that medical writing appears credible and communicates effectively with its audience.
- Queries to authors should be polite yet concise. Unnecessary querying should be avoided.

- Editing for mechanics includes checking punctuation, grammar, spelling (including irregular plurals), abbreviations, and capitalization.
- Medical copyediting includes attention to word usage, the use of eponyms and toponyms, and the use of unbiased, respectful wording.
- Although medical editors are not expected to be mathematicians, they should be alert for basic problems in number use and statistics.
- Copyediting also includes editing for consistency with a publication's style (for example, the conventions followed regarding number format, punctuation, and reference format).
- Style sheets are important for keeping track of the conventions being followed in an editing project and otherwise maintaining consistency in it.
- Copyediting can include editing tables and providing editorial feedback on figures.

· EXERCISE ·

Some Sentences to Copyedit

Please copyedit the following sentences. Do not make any other changes. AMA style should be followed insofar as feasible.

1. Of the 47 diabetics confined to wheelchairs, 23 (48.9361 %) utilized Ibuprofen.
2. According to HIPPA, PA's should not reveal such information about the cases they treat.
3. This 67-year old female with Parkinson's Disease also suffered from Irritable Bowel Syndrome (IBS), which lead her to consult our clinic.
4. Symptoms of this disease include: fever, fatigue and a distinctive rash.
5. This year, 4 students will report on Staphylococcus Aureus during the unit on preventative medicine.
6. 274 black patients met all the inclusion criterion for the study.
7. Her main mentor, Dr. Li helped her design the research and her writing-instructor helped her edit the resulting paper.
8. Waiting for the bus, his foot began to ache, his skin began to itch, and twitching of his ears started.

9. The day before the procedure; you should only consume clear liquids such as lemon-lime gateraid.
10. Because this test often fails to detect cases, researchers at the National Institute of Health [NEH] are trying to device one with greater specificity.

· 5 ·

Substantive Editing

EDITING FOR CONTENT AND ORGANIZATION

As discussed in the previous chapter, copyediting mainly entails ensuring that mechanics such as grammar, spelling, and punctuation are correct and that appropriate stylistic conventions are followed. However, editing also can entail evaluating and improving content and organization. Editing that addresses these latter aspects is known as *substantive editing*. To use a medical analogy: Whereas copyediting helps ensure that the skin of a document is unblemished, substantive editing helps ensure that the skeleton of the document is sound, that the muscle is appropriately robust, and that all needed organs are present and functional.

Substantive editing and copyediting are not mutually exclusive. Sometimes the final editing of a document incorporates both. Sometimes an early draft of a document undergoes mainly substantive editing, and later the finished version is copyedited. Sometimes, alternating between copyediting and substantive editing can work well: Problems with content or organization may become apparent once copyediting has clarified meaning, and substantive changes may necessitate further copyediting.

The current chapter focuses on substantive editing of medical writing. First it discusses the scope of substantive editing. Then it addresses substantively editing journal articles reporting medical research. Guidance also is provided on substantively editing other types of medical writing, such as case reports, news reports, and grant proposals. The chapter also introduces published guidelines for reporting specific types of medical research and discusses using them to help guide substantive editing.

Substantive Editing: Scope and Rationale

No matter how polished a piece of medical writing may be, it is unlikely to succeed fully if its structure is unsound, if content is incorrect or missing or superfluous, or if reasoning in it is flawed. Therefore, substantive editing can be important for medical writing. Given its focus, substantive editing helps ensure the validity of the medical literature as a basis for further research. It also helps ensure the validity of this literature as a basis for application, such as in clinical practice or in public health policy. Finally, it helps ensure readability, comprehensibility, and persuasiveness—all of which are important for maximal impact.

A copyeditor asks mainly "Is the document mechanically correct and consistent with the publisher's style?" In contrast, a substantive editor asks largely "Does the document have the appropriate content and structure, and does everything make sense?" Substantive editing can occur before or after submission of a document. Before submission, an editor at the author's institution or a freelance editor may substantively edit journal articles, grant proposals, book manuscripts, and other materials. Once a journal article or book manuscript is accepted, an editor on the publisher's staff or a freelance or contract editor engaged by the publisher may do editing with substantive components.

Whatever the type of document, substantive editing tends to address some core questions. One is *completeness*: Does all the needed content seem to be present? If not, what appears to be missing? Another is *focus*: Is all the content relevant? If not, what seems to deserve deletion? A third category is *organization*: For example, have the relevant structural conventions been followed? If not, what changes should be made to comply with these conventions? Also, at various levels, does the structure make sense? For example, are events presented chronologically when warranted, do paragraphs start with strong topic sentences, and do items in a list appear in a logical order? A fourth category regards *logic* in other respects: In particular, is each conclusion consistent with the evidence presented? Finally, substantive editing may include checking for *ethics*: For example, have conflicts of interest been disclosed if required, and have lapses in confidentiality been avoided? More generally, substantive editing also entails being alert for anything that appears suspicious—for instance, a date that seems unlikely, a size that seems implausible, or a definition that seems incorrect.

Often, resolving substantive problems entails querying authors, so they can address the problem or indicate how the editor should do so. Examples of queries corresponding to the categories noted above are the following:

COMPLETENESS

- "According to the provided guidelines, this section also should specify the method of randomization. I suggest adding this content."
- "Typically, a paragraph on limitations of the study appears at approximately this point in the discussion section. Adding such a paragraph seems advisable."

FOCUS

- "It appears unclear why the material I've highlighted is included. I suggest either deleting it or making explicit its relationship to the other content."
- "The section on historical perspectives seems disproportionately long for use in a chapter of this type. Perhaps consider condensing it. Maybe some of the material could appear in an appendix or be published as a historical essay."

ORGANIZATION

- "It was unclear to me why the countries were listed in this order. Perhaps list them alphabetically. Or if they were listed according to some other principle (for example, from earliest to latest to report cases), I suggest specifying it."
- "This paragraph on the experimental protocol seems rather long and difficult to follow. A flowchart or table might be more effective. If you would like, I could draft one to consider."

LOGIC

- "In discussing the correlation that this study found between participation in collegiate sports and subsequent high grades in medical school surgery clerkships, it is stated that therefore premedical students should engage in collegiate sports. However, is the relationship necessarily causal? Could the same traits (such as physical coordination and a team orientation) that lead students

to take part in collegiate sports also contribute to success in surgery clerkships? Perhaps also discuss the latter possibility."
- "Here it is stated that most of the patients reported relief of the symptom. However, the results section states that 189 of the 400 patients did so. Please reword accordingly, for example by changing 'most' to 'almost half.'"

ETHICS
- "I see that in this report the patients are identified by their initials. This approach does not sufficiently conceal their identity. I suggest identifying the patients as Patient 1, Patient 2, etc."
- "I noticed that this diagram was the same as in the textbook that was cited. The diagram doesn't seem to have a source line. Was permission to use this diagram obtained? If so, was wording for a source line specified?"

OTHER
- "Here it is said that the catheter was 2.5 km wide. I wonder whether 'km' was a typo. Was another unit, such as mm, meant? If so, please specify."
- "More recent rates in this regard have now been posted at ____. I suggest using the more recent rates."

A question that sometimes arises is whether you can substantively edit a document without being an expert on the subject being addressed. Even without subject-matter expertise, you can contribute much, for example by attending to the internal logic of the writing and being aware of conventions such as those noted later in this chapter. However, subject-matter knowledge can help you to edit more thoroughly, accurately, and efficiently. An example encountered: An author wrote that follow-up examinations after an abnormal Pap test may include colonoscopy. The editor correctly concluded that the author meant *colposcopy* (viewing of the vagina and cervix with a magnifying instrument), not *colonoscopy* (viewing of the colon via a specialized long tube).

An editor's medical knowledge may come from education, for example in biomedical science or a health profession. It also can come from experience, including work in medically related settings and even being a patient or a patient's friend or family member. Such knowledge also can come from background reading (and viewing) and from discussing the subject at hand, for instance with the author or fellow editors. And the experience you gain as a medical editor can contribute greatly to your fund of knowledge and thus help prepare you for future substantive editing.

Editing Journal Articles Reporting Research

Journal articles reporting medical research usually appear in the IMRAD format (introduction, methods, results, and discussion), which is commonly used for scientific papers. Occasionally, they appear in variants of this format. For example, some journals publish papers having a combined results and discussion section, with results and discussion interspersed. And some journals, especially in basic science, place the methods section last. Having standard structures for scientific papers and other types of journal articles helps authors—and editors—ensure that all needed content is present, that the article is logically structured, and that content is accessibly presented. Likewise, having standard, familiar structures for articles helps readers know where in an article to find various types of information.

Like other editing, substantively editing a journal article can benefit from following a basic routine. Steps may include learning (or learning more) about the topic, identifying the target journal and its requirements, starting a style sheet and then developing it further as the editing progresses, reading the article as a whole for an overview, editing sections in a preferred order, reviewing the editing from beginning to end of the paper to ensure consistency and coherence, and reviewing the title and abstract a final time to make sure that they accurately represent the content. Reviewing a hard copy of the manuscript at one or more stages can aid in getting a sense of the whole and in detecting problems difficult to notice onscreen.

The amount of learning about the topic tends to distinguish substantive editing from copyediting, as more understanding of the content is beneficial. Such learning may be iterative, including initially orienting oneself to the topic and then looking items up as they arise. Avoid, however, the trap of trying to become an expert on the subject (if you are not one already). You are not a peer reviewer or fact checker, and the author has ultimate responsibility for the content. In general, your goal should be to grasp the content sufficiently to follow the story and the reasoning and to query the author when clues exist that revisions in content may be warranted.

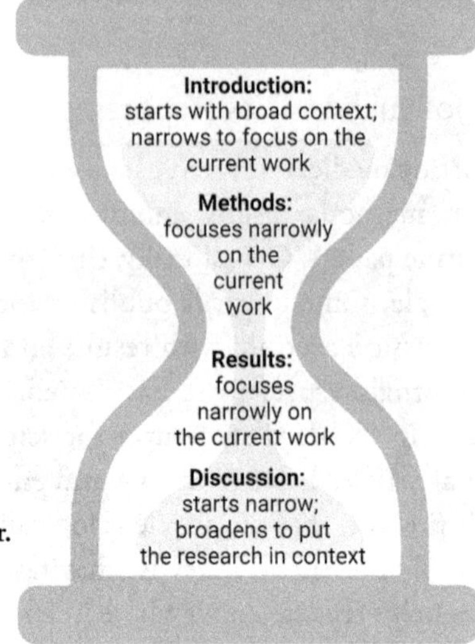

Created in BioRender. Gastel, B. (2024) https://BioRender.com/e90r606.

So, how might you gain some familiarity with a medical topic on which you will edit a journal article? Lay-oriented materials on the subject—for example, those accessed through the National Institutes of Health meta-resource MedlinePlus (https://medlineplus.gov/)—can be a fine start. So can textbook chapters and review articles; in the biomedical literature database PubMed (https://pubmed.ncbi.nlm.nih.gov/), you can search specifically for review articles. Looking at articles cited in the manuscript also can help in understanding the content and knowing norms for presenting it. And don't neglect human sources. A discussion with the author can orient you to content and identify aspects of the paper on which the author would especially like editorial input.

In considering the substance of an IMRAD-style journal article, it can help to envision such an article as a story answering a series of four questions. In brief, the introduction should address "What question was the research meant to answer?" The methods section should address "How did the researchers try to answer it?" The results section should address "What did the researchers find?" And the discussion should address "What does it mean?" It also can be helpful to envision the shape of a scientific paper as an hourglass—with the introduction beginning with broad background and then narrowing down to the research question, the methods and results sections focusing tightly on the present research, and then the discussion broadening out to put the findings in context.

Of course, a paper in IMRAD format also contains more than IMRAD. It normally starts with a title, author list, and abstract. And it normally ends with acknowledgments and references. In some journals, articles reporting research also have other sections, such as a bulleted list of take-home points for clinicians. The following are some questions to consider when substantively editing an IMRAD-type article.

TITLE

The title is the most widely read part of a journal article. It is crucial in literature searching. And readers use it to decide whether to read further. Therefore, it deserves especially careful editing. For consistency with the rest of the paper, it should receive a final edit after the rest of the paper is edited. A preliminary edit earlier can be helpful as well.

The key question to ask is "Does the title accurately capture the essence of the paper?" Although a cute or cryptic title might suit a blog post, editorial, or poster presentation, the title of a journal article presenting research should be informative and straightforward. If it does not seem informative enough, or if it seems unclear or potentially misleading, try to propose one or more alternative titles that can at least be starting points for revision.

Other questions to consider include "Does the title comply with the journal's requirements?" For example, some journals limit the number of words or characters in titles. And journals vary as to whether they accept titles that are worded as questions (such as "Does Drug X Alleviate Condition Y?"), that are worded as sentences ("Drug X Alleviates Condition Y"), or that have parts separated by colons ("Condition Y: Alleviation by Drug X"), rather than more conventionally structured titles ("Effect of Drug X on Condition Y"). Thus, substantive editing can include condensing a title to meet length restrictions and restructuring titles to suit the target journal.

It also can be relevant to ask, "Does the title follow relevant conventions or guidelines, if any, regarding content?" For example, the CONSORT guidelines (https://www.equator-network.org/reporting-guidelines/consort/), which regard journal articles reporting randomized trials, say the title should identify the research as a randomized trial. And more generally, some journals request that the title state the study design (for example, "Habit A as a Risk Factor for Disease B: A Case-Control Study" or "Habit A as a Risk Factor for Disease B: A Longitudinal Study"). If a title lacks information of a type requested, a substantive editor should indicate what is missing and, if feasible, propose a revised title.

Journals sometimes request *running titles*—in other words, shortened titles that appear at the tops of pages—and indicate the number of characters allowed. A substantive editor may check whether a running title is provided if required, see whether a given running title seems suitable, and, if relevant, draft a running title or propose a revised running title. For example, if a title is "Effects of Regimen XYZ on P, Q, and R in College Students with Condition ABC of More Than 2 Years' Duration: A Randomized Controlled Trial" (138 characters, including spaces) but the journal requests a running title of no more than 50 characters, including spaces, one possibility to propose would be "Effects of Regimen XYZ in Long-Term Condition ABC" (49 characters, including spaces).

AUTHORS

Substantive editing can include helping to ensure that the author list contains the appropriate names. It also can include helping to ensure that, if the target journal requests, the contributions of authors and relevant others are specified.

Those with major intellectual contributions to the research should be listed as authors. Many medical journals follow the International Committee of Medical Journal Editors recommendations (https://www.icmje.org/recommendations/browse/roles-and-responsibilities/defining-the-role-of-authors-and-contributors.html), which state that to qualify for authorship, an individual should meet all four criteria stated as follows:

- Substantial contributions to the conception or design of the work; or the acquisition, analysis, or interpretation of data for the work; AND
- Drafting the work or revising it critically for important intellectual content; AND
- Final approval of the version to be published; AND
- Agreement to be accountable for all aspects of the work in ensuring that questions related to the accuracy or integrity of any part of the work are appropriately investigated and resolved.

Regardless of whether a journal uses these criteria or somewhat different ones, the author list should include all those, and only those, who qualify. Individuals should not be excluded because, for example, they are students or technicians rather than contributors of higher rank. Likewise, a paper should not list people who contributed little or nothing to the research but are being included to advance their careers, to show appreciation of general support, or to add prestige.

Some journals also require submissions to state who contributed what to the work. Listed contributors should include not only individuals whose contributions qualify them to be authors but also others, if any, who contributed—for example, those who collected data but did not play other roles, who provided advice, or (yes!) who substantively edited the manuscript. Some journals specify wording to use for contributor roles. A list of contributor roles appears in CRediT (the Contributor Role Taxonomy; https://credit.niso.org/).

Responsibility for ensuring that the appropriate people are listed as authors (and, if relevant, as contributors) is primarily the main authors'. However, substantive editing can include flagging possible discrepancies in this regard. For example, if listed contributions seem likely to qualify someone for authorship but the person is not listed as an author, the editor should ask about the potential omission. Or if someone listed as an author has no contributions listed, the editor should query. Likewise, if the research seems likely to have involved a statistician but one is not listed as an author or contributor, it can be worth asking whether such an individual should be identified. In short: In author lists, as in the body of the paper, substantive editing does not entail verifying all facts but rather identifying content that may merit authors' checking.

ABSTRACT AND KEYWORDS

An abstract summarizes a paper. Its main function is to help readers determine whether to read the entire paper. Even if a paper is not widely accessible, the abstract tends to be openly available, for example through PubMed. Thus, the abstract tends to be the most read part of a paper other than the title. Given the role and wide availability of an abstract, ensuring its accuracy and readability is especially important.

Normally, the abstract appears before the body of the paper and is organized like the paper (for example, in IMRAD format). Some medical journals use *structured abstracts*—that is, abstracts containing standardized headings, such as "Context," "Methods," "Results," and "Conclusions." Others have abstracts that are organized in this way but do not include headings. Sometimes journals with structured abstracts have somewhat different sets of headings for papers reporting different types of research. Journals normally have word limits for abstracts; often, the limit is 250 words (approximately the equivalent of one double-spaced page). Thus, abstracts must be informative but concise.

Substantive editing includes ensuring that the content of the abstract is consistent with that of the body of the paper. It also includes helping to ensure that the key content is indeed present and that superfluous details are not. In addition, it includes helping to ensure that, regardless of whether the abstract is structured or unstructured, the abstract is suitably organized. It also entails making sure that the abstract makes sense on its own, without reading the rest of the paper; for example, abbreviations should be defined, results should be stated only if corresponding methods are mentioned, and references normally should not be cited. Especially given word limits, editing an abstract also includes editing for conciseness.

Traditionally, abstracts of journal articles reporting medical research have not contained figures and tables. However, some medical journals now present the main message of at least some papers pictorially through *visual abstracts* (Ibrahim 2024) or *graphical abstracts*. The two terms often are used interchangeably, but sometimes the former denotes a three-panel format but the latter a one-panel format (Scott 2019). For a substantive editor, reviewing such an abstract can include (in addition to checking whether the journal's instructions for visual or graphical abstracts were followed) seeing whether the visuals seem to accurately represent the content of the paper; seeing whether they appear easy to follow; checking the text for accuracy, clarity, and mechanics—and, if warranted, proposing revisions.

Because the abstract must represent the content of the paper, it should undergo final editing after the rest of the paper is finalized. At that point, any changes in the paper's content will have been made. And at that point, the substantive editor will understand the paper most fully. However, preliminary editing of abstracts early on can serve as useful context for editing the rest of the paper. Indeed, several editorial rounds at different stages can be most effective in editing an abstract.

In some journals, a list of several *keywords* follows the abstract. Keywords are terms that indicate the main topics of an article, much as terms in an index would. Substantive editing can include checking whether keywords are included if the journal requires them and, if they are present, seeing whether they seem suitable. Some journals request that the number of keywords be within a given range. Some also have other requirements, such as that the terms come from a specified list or that the keywords not be terms used in the title, which already are clear choices for use in indexing or literature searching. Thus, the substantive editor should check the journal's instructions to authors for any requirements regarding keywords. If a list of keywords should be added or if it seems that any keywords should be added, deleted, or replaced, presenting the suggestions in a query is in order.

THE INTRODUCTION

The introduction should provide context for understanding and appreciating the rest of the paper. It also should identify the question (or questions) or the hypothesis (or hypotheses) that the research addressed. Typically, the introduction should resemble a funnel, proceeding from broad to narrow. Accordingly, it generally should start by providing background on the topic, next present highlights of relevant previous research, then identify a relevant gap in the knowledge, and then specify what the research was accordingly intended to answer. A general statement of the approach taken may follow. In some journals, the main finding may also be stated, foreshadowing content later in the paper.

Different journals, or different types of journals, tend to have introductions of different lengths. In medical journals, reports of original research tend to have fairly short introductions, ranging from one paragraph to several paragraphs. In contrast, some social science journals publishing medically oriented articles and some nursing journals routinely run long introductions containing extensive reviews of the literature. Seeing whether an introduction falls within the usual length range for the target journal, and suggesting condensation or expansion if it does not, can be part of substantive editing.

Substantive editing of an introduction also can include assessing whether the introduction seems suited for the target audience. For example, if an article in a specialized research area is being submitted to a general medical journal, the authors may need to add basic background, define some key terms, and explain some underlying concepts. If, however, the article is being submitted to a specialized journal in the authors' research area, a substantive editor might well advise the authors to remove or condense some material that is relatively elementary. As a representative of the readership, a substantive editor can counsel the authors in such regards.

In addition, substantively editing an introduction entails checking whether it contains the basic elements and presents them in a logical order, such as the funnel structure. Major questions to consider include the following: Does the opening demonstrate the importance of the subject? For example, if an article regards a given disease, are sufficient statistics presented, if relevant, on its incidence, prevalence, and economic impact? Is the gap in previous research made apparent? Is the purpose of the research clearly defined, either through one or more research questions or hypotheses or through a statement such as "In order to determine . . ."?

Functions of the introduction also can include helping to show the originality, novelty, and priority of the research being reported in the paper. Sometimes, manuscripts state unequivocally that something has not been reported before or proclaim definitively that the current research is the first in some regard. Such statements may be true, but they cannot be proven; perhaps, for instance, similar findings from another group still are undergoing publication or were reported in an obscure venue. Thus, substantive editing can include, for example, suggesting that "this approach has not been previously evaluated in this condition" be revised to read "review of the literature has not disclosed previous evaluation of this approach in this condition." Likewise, such editing can include recommending that the authors change "We are the first to report" to wording such as "We appear to be the first to report."

THE METHODS SECTION

The methods section serves two functions. First, it provides the information needed for others to replicate the research or conduct analogous research. Second, it allows others to evaluate the research, both to assess its quality and to consider its broader applicability. Information from which to determine broader applicability can be especially important in reports of medical research, because many medical readers want to know whether the findings appear applicable to the patients or populations they serve. For example, if a study was done in female college athletes, a physician might wonder about its applicability to a 90-year-old male patient; a study in retired men might be more clearly applicable.

On a macro level, substantive editing of a methods section can include helping to ensure that all needed types of content are present. Depending in part on the target journal and the type of research, the methods may begin with an overview of the research design. If such an overview is present, it should be checked for consistency with what follows. If it is not present and might be appropriate and useful, adding it may be suggested. Examples of other types of content that may need to be specified include populations or organisms studied, laboratory methods used, and statistical methods employed. In some journals, the methods section may include subheadings to designate different types of content; if such subheadings could be useful but are not present, they can be suggested. If methods sections contain figures—such as flowcharts, diagrams, maps, or timelines—or tables, their content and crafting should be assessed. And if adding any such items could aid in communicating the methods, they may be suggested.

Research on humans or animals must be approved beforehand by an appropriate group (an *institutional review board*, or IRB, in the former case or an *institutional animal care and use committee*, or IACUC, in the latter). Only if such approvals have been obtained will a journal consider publishing the research. Commonly, documentation of the approval appears in the methods section. If such information appears to be needed but missing, an editor should query.

The scope of the methods section should be consistent with that of the results section. Only if corresponding results are reported should a given method be noted. Likewise, for every result reported, it should be clear how that result was obtained. Authors should be informed of any inconsistencies in this regard.

On the micro level, the methods section should contain sufficient detail for both replication and evaluation. For example: What mouse strain was used, and from what breeder? What were the demographics (age, sex, etc.) of the patients? How large were the groups studied, and how was the sample size determined? Were the groups' identities (such as experimental group and control group) concealed, and if so, how? What was the manufacturer of the drug? What company made the reagent, and what were the manufacturer and model of the equipment? How was the assay done? If details regarding the assay do not appear in the current paper, where have they been published? What statistical software package was used? Journals can differ somewhat among themselves in how much detail they customarily include about methods. If in doubt, looking at reports of analogous research in the target journal can help; if the current level of detail seems to differ markedly, alerting the author to the difference can be advisable.

THE RESULTS SECTION

The results—in other words, what the researchers found—form the core of the paper. Like other parts of the paper, the results section should be logically organized. For some research, presenting findings chronologically, in the order in which they were obtained, makes most sense. In other instances, starting with the most important result and progressing to the least important is most appropriate. For some types of research, a customary order of presentation exists; for instance, in reporting on a case series, it is customary to begin with pertinent aspects of the medical histories, then describe the physical findings in the group of patients, and then summarize laboratory findings—rather than, for example, starting with laboratory findings. If the organization of a results section seems less than ideal, substantive editing can include improving the organization or suggesting improvements.

Results sections of medical papers usually contain tables, figures, or both. Substantive editing includes helping to ensure that each table or figure makes sense, provides the needed information, does not include superfluous information (such as a column of all zeroes, which generally can be replaced by a footnote or other text or deleted), and is well designed. The editing also includes ensuring that each table or figure is mentioned at the relevant point(s) in the text, that the main point of each table or figure is noted in the text, and that, if doing so appears useful, the text states key data from the figure or table. The text should not, however, repeat in detail the content of a table or figure. When this common problem occurs, substantive editing includes reducing the redundancy or guiding the author in doing so.

Beyond considering the existing tables and figures, substantive editing can include considering whether any tables or figures should be added. For example, would any information currently in the text be better conveyed by a table or figure? Would the content of a current table be better communicated in a figure, or vice versa? Do any tables or figures contribute so little that perhaps they should be deleted? Might any be worth dividing or combining? If the journal posts supplementary tables and figures, should anything be moved to or from this category?

The results section is the main place statistics appear. A substantive editor is not expected to be a statistician, but statistical literacy can strengthen substantive editing. If, given your understanding, something in the manuscript seems statistically implausible, it should be queried. Likewise, if statistical information seems to be missing—for example, if differences are said to be statistically significant but the paper seems not to provide support such as *P* values or confidence intervals—the author should be alerted.

Often, the results section of a draft contains too many trees but too little forest. The data abound, but the patterns are not apparent enough. Two groups of authors seem especially prone to this difficulty. One consists of early-career authors who feel a need to include every hard-won bit of data or who still are developing their sense of focus. Another such group consists of authors who are writing papers for US or other Western journals but whose cultural traditions favor expression that is much more indirect than suits these journals. For these groups of authors and some others, a substantive editor can help both in dealing with the trees and in enhancing the forest. The editor can help manage the trees through means such as summarizing or condensing data, proposing use of representative rather than exhaustive data, and identifying tangential data for the author to consider deleting. And the editor can help display the forest more distinctly by revising paragraphs so they begin with strong topic sentences and then contain data in support of them. Such revisions can help the authors present their results clearly and thus tell their story persuasively.

THE DISCUSSION

The discussion section tends to be especially difficult for authors to write, as there is more choice of content than elsewhere in the paper. Accordingly, substantive editors can be of particular help in refining this section.

In keeping with the hourglass format for scientific papers, the discussion should begin by focusing narrowly on the current findings, and it should then place them in progressively broader contexts. Typically, it should start with a brief recap of the main finding(s) of the research. Doing so serves two main functions. First, it reminds readers of what will be discussed. Second, not everyone reads the parts of a scientific paper in the order in which they appear. Therefore, each component should be understandable on its own. Summarizing the findings orients readers who jump to the discussion. As a substantive editor, check whether such a recap of the main findings is present. If it is missing, suggest adding it, and perhaps propose wording for it. If it is present, ensure that it is consistent with the material in previous sections and that it is well focused, clear, and concise.

The introduction should have explicitly or implicitly stated one or more research questions or hypotheses. Early in the discussion, these questions or hypotheses should be addressed. For example, if the research question was "Does intervention A help prevent condition B?" (or the hypothesis was "Intervention A helps prevent condition B."), the discussion should contain a statement such as (depending on the results) "Our findings indicate that intervention A helps prevent condition B," "Our findings indicate that intervention A does not help prevent condition B," or "It is unclear from our findings whether intervention A helps prevent condition B." Too often, the manuscript does not directly address the main question or hypothesis or addresses something different from what was asked (for example, by focusing on an interesting side effect of A without saying whether A seems to help prevent B). A substantive editor should check whether each research question or hypothesis is explicitly addressed; if it is not addressed, recommend doing so. If there was only one main question or hypothesis, the discussion may then proceed to putting the answer in context. If more than one research question or hypothesis was explored, an alternative to addressing them all before moving to broader discussion is to put the answer to each in context before addressing the next.

Of course, the answers must be consistent with the evidence. Sometimes authors overstate findings or generalize more broadly than the data can safely allow. If the conclusions seem to overstep the data, tactfully note the possibility, and perhaps propose more cautious wording. Do the findings actually *prove*? Or do they *indicate* or perhaps *suggest*? Can the findings confidently be generalized to other populations? Or should some uncertainty be noted in that regard?

If the findings contained discrepancies (for example, if the findings in one subgroup ran counter to the findings in the group as a whole), early in the discussion can be a good place to address them. Here, the authors may remind readers of the discrepancies, state possible reasons for them, note possible effects (if any) on the conclusions, and, if warranted, say how the discrepancies might be addressed in future research. If substantial discrepancies exist but have not been discussed, a substantive editor may recommend addressing them. If discrepancies are indeed addressed, a substantive editor can help ensure that their discussion appears complete, logical, and clear.

As the hourglass broadens, the paper should place the findings in the context of previously published research. How are the findings consistent with those previously reported? How, if at all, do they differ from previous findings, and why might the differences have occurred? What do the current findings add to medical knowledge? Substantive editing can include helping to ensure that such questions are addressed. It can also help ensure that this aspect of the discussion is thorough yet focused and that it is logical and clear.

As the discussion broadens still further, it tends to focus next on implications, applications, or both. Depending on the type of research, examples of questions that may be addressed include the following: What do the findings tell us about basic biomedical mechanisms? Do the findings support current models or theories, refute them, or suggest modifications of them? What recommendations do the findings favor regarding patient care? What do the findings suggest regarding public health policy? Substantive editing can include helping to ensure that relevant such questions are indeed addressed, that the authors are neither too restrained nor too sweeping in discussing implications and applications, and that the reasoning appears valid and easy to follow.

Near the end, the discussion customarily addresses limitations of the research. In medical research, examples of common limitations include relatively small sample size, limited diversity of participants studied, sizeable numbers of dropouts from the study, limited length of follow-up, and limitations of laboratory procedures. Some authors hesitate to mention limitations, for fear that doing so would prevent a journal from accepting their paper or would diminish the impact of their paper. However, discussing limitations is the norm, and journals and readers may consider failure to do so a deficiency. Indeed, identifying limitations and their implications is part of being transparent about research. Also, if authors do not note the limitations themselves, peer reviewers or readers may do so—perhaps harshly. Further, if authors state the limitations themselves, they themselves can discuss the implications, which may turn out to be minor. Also, noting limitations can lead smoothly into presenting suggestions for further research. Substantive editing can include helping to ensure that a limitations section is present and sound.

As well as noting limitations of the research, a discussion section may note strengths. Sometimes authors consider it immodest to do so. However, doing so can help show that the paper adds markedly to the literature. Noting strengths can especially help if the findings are not very novel but the research had other pluses. For example, if the findings resembled those of an earlier study but the methods were more robust and thus the conclusions are more definitive, that fact may be worth stating. Substantive editing may include advising authors on whether—and if so, how—to note strengths of the study. Sometimes, information on strengths can fit well with that on limitations. In other instances, the information may fit well elsewhere in the discussion section, for example in the section comparing the current study and earlier ones.

Some papers reporting medical research end with a freestanding section titled Conclusions. Commonly, however, the last paragraph of the discussion serves as the conclusion. This paragraph is likely to state, in a few sentences, what was done, what was found, and what the take-home message is. Because this paragraph comes last, it can be especially impactful. Also, some readers read it first, to decide whether to read more of the paper. For both reasons, this paragraph can deserve especially careful editing, both for accuracy and for clarity and readability.

Authors often are unsure what to include in the discussion section. Therefore, frequently this part of the manuscript either is underdeveloped and too short or is too long and rambling. Substantive editing of the discussion therefore tends to include considering its scope and focus. When editors can work with authors early in the writing process, they can guide them on what to include and how much detail to provide. Looking at the discussion sections of analogous papers in the intended journal can guide authors and editors on how extensive the section should be.

ACKNOWLEDGMENTS

The acknowledgments section is the place mainly for authors to identify, and express appreciation of, people's contributions that do not qualify for authorship but nevertheless aided in the research or its publication. Examples of the many types of help that may be acknowledged include gathering data, sharing materials or equipment, providing basic statistical assistance, supplying feedback on drafts, and editing the manuscript before submission. In addition, medical articles may acknowledge others such as health care professionals who referred patients to participate in the study and, though not by name, the patients or other participants who were studied.

In a journal article, only professionally related contributions should be acknowledged. Unlike in a master's thesis or doctoral dissertation, authors should not thank their parents and partners and friends for their support, their dogs and cats and ferrets for their loyalty, and the local coffee shop for providing the caffeine needed to power the endeavor.

Typically, the wording of acknowledgments should be simple and straightforward. For example, it may read "We thank Susie Sophomore for persistent and precise pipetting, Nell Numerate for statistical help, and Will Wordsmith for editorial assistance." Flowery accolades should be left for theses and dissertations and perhaps for the party celebrating the paper's publication.

In some journals, the acknowledgments section is the place to identify the source, or sources, of financial support for the research (or to say there was no outside financial support). In other journals, such identification appears elsewhere, such as in a footnote. Some funding sources, such as government agencies and private foundations, require that papers reporting research that they funded include such identification. Likewise, journals typically require it. Even when funding sources or others do not require such disclosure, it is highly advisable for transparency and therefore should be present.

Typically, acknowledgments sections require little substantive editing. However, a substantive editor may suggest additions to or deletions from the list of those acknowledged, in keeping with principles noted in this section, and they may make copyeditorial revisions. Likewise, substantive editors should ensure that sources of funding are disclosed in the acknowledgments or elsewhere.

REFERENCES

Editing the reference list of a scientific paper tends to be at least mainly copyediting. However, some aspects can merit a substantive editor's attention. One item to notice is whether the reference list seems up-to-date. Sometimes, for example, the authors completed the research months or more ago and have not updated their literature search. If a reference list lacks recent references, a substantive editor may ask the authors whether updating is needed. At the other extreme, sometimes the list includes only recent references, although older references also might warrant inclusion. Here too, a substantive editor may suggest checking whether the literature has been well enough reviewed. In addition, substantive editing includes being attuned to the credibility of references. For example, an article in a reputable journal generally is valid to cite; an article in Wikipedia generally is not. If a cited source seems to have questionable credibility, a query can be advisable.

The balance of references also can be worth considering. Sometimes a manuscript cites multiple references by its own authors. Doing so can be valid, because often the current research builds on the authors' earlier research. However, because researchers, institutions, and journals sometimes use citation counts as measures of prominence, authors sometimes cite their own work excessively, in a conscious or unconscious attempt to increase their citations in the literature. If some self-citations do not seem very relevant, a query may be in order. Likewise, if a work by others is relevant, the authors should not neglect to cite it even if they dislike its authors or are competitors.

Throughout the paper, help ensure that references are cited whenever advisable. For example: In the introduction, are references cited sufficiently when providing background for the current research? In the methods section, are they cited for specialized techniques referred to? And in the discussion, are they cited enough when interpreting results and placing them in context? (Because the results section reports only the current findings, rarely if ever should references appear in it.) In places where adding references seems advisable, query to propose considering doing so. Likewise, if some citations seem superfluous—for example, if they just seem to support common knowledge in the readers' field—suggest considering their deletion.

Finally, the total number of references can be a consideration. Some journals limit the number of references per paper. If so, a substantive editor may aid in ensuring that the most relevant references are cited. In any case, substantive editing can include helping the authors ensure that the extent of citation is within the norms for the authors' discipline and the intended journal.

A checklist can aid in editing journal articles in the IMRAD format. Such a checklist accompanies this chapter. Feel free to use it as is or modify it to serve you best.

Editing Journal Articles in the IMRAD Format: Some Questions to Ask

TITLE

- Does the title accurately capture the essence of the paper?
- Does the title comply with the journal's requirements (for example, regarding length)?
- Does the title follow relevant conventions or guidelines, if any?

AUTHORS

- Do all those listed qualify for authorship?
- Has anyone been left out?
- If applicable, have the contributions of authors and relevant others been identified?

ABSTRACT

- Is the abstract suitably organized ("mini-IMRAD")?
- If a structured abstract is required, is one provided, and are the correct headings used?
- If a graphical abstract is requested, is one provided?
- Is any content missing or superfluous?
- Is the abstract consistent with the rest of the paper?

INTRODUCTION

- Does the introduction suit the audience?
- Does the length of the introduction suit the journal?
- Is the introduction suitably structured (typically, broad to narrow)?

METHODS

- If warranted, is there an overview of the research design?
- If the research was on humans or animals, are the needed approvals noted?
- Are all methods described?
- Are the descriptions of methods suitably detailed?
- If relevant, are items such as subheadings, tables, and figures used?

RESULTS

- Do the results match the purpose and methods?
- Are the results presented in appropriate detail?
- Are the results organized logically and in keeping with relevant conventions and guidelines?
- Are the tables and figures, if any, suitable?
- Does the text identify key points from tables and figures but avoid excessive redundancy with them?

DISCUSSION

- Does the discussion answer the question(s) asked?
- Are the conclusions consistent with the evidence?
- Are the findings placed in the context of the previous literature?
- If appropriate, are implications and applications discussed?
- Does the discussion address limitations (and possible strengths)?
- Is the discussion reasonably structured (typically, narrow to broad)?
- Is the discussion an appropriate length?
- If there's not a separate conclusions section, does the discussion sum up?

ACKNOWLEDGMENTS

- Are all those deserving acknowledgment acknowledged?
- Does the list include anyone inappropriate to acknowledge?
- Are funding sources acknowledged, either here or in another suitable location?

REFERENCES

- Have all listed references been cited in the text?
- Do all cited references appear in the reference list?
- Does the list include suitably recent references?
- Does the list include older references where warranted?
- Do credible sources seem to have been cited?
- Has excessive self-citation been avoided?
- Are all references in the proper format?

Editing Other Main Types of Journal Articles

In addition to scientific papers presenting research, medical journals often include other content. Examples include review articles summarizing and integrating information from multiple published studies, case reports describing and analyzing noteworthy clinical cases, editorials and other commentary placing research in context or advocating standpoints in health policy or other realms, letters to the editor commenting on work published in the journal, and even literary work on medical themes. Substantive editors may especially be called on to edit review articles and case reports before or after submission. Guidance in editing these two genres follows.

REVIEW ARTICLES

Review articles summarize and integrate the literature on given topics. Typically, they integrate knowledge from many journal articles. Because they efficiently provide overviews, they are popular with various groups of medical readers—including researchers seeking to keep up with developments or broaden their knowledge, graduate students gaining a foundation in the field, health professionals needing to stay up-to-date, health-professional students establishing their knowledge base, and sometimes patients and those holding them dear. Because many readers rely on review articles to be authoritative, authors of medical review articles have a serious responsibility to ensure that these articles are informative, accurate, balanced, and clear. Substantive editing of medical review articles supports authors in such regards.

Review articles have a traditional structure but also may follow an IMRAD-like format. The traditional structure resembles that of a book chapter, with sections on various subtopics. For example, a review article on a disease might include sections on signs and symptoms, cause and disease mechanism, diagnosis, treatment, prognosis, and future research directions. In contrast, an IMRAD-type review article commonly includes an introduction providing context and defining the purpose of the review, a methods section describing how the literature was searched and analyzed, a results section presenting the findings of the search, and a discussion interpreting those findings. Traditional review articles, sometimes known as narrative reviews, tend to be well suited for providing overviews of broad topics; IMRAD-style reviews tend to excel at addressing well-focused questions (for example, whether, according to the various studies done, a given treatment is effective in a given condition). A related type of article is a meta-analysis, in which quantitative findings from various studies are combined, in search of a conclusion more robust than those of individual studies. Librarians and others have devised classifications of review articles (for example, Grant and Booth 2009); categories include scoping reviews (which provide preliminary assessments of the literature), systematic reviews (so called because of their methodical approach), and state-of-the-art reviews (which focus largely on current matters). Familiarity with such categories and the expectations for them can aid in substantive editing.

For traditional review articles, some questions to address in substantive editing are the following:

- Is the overall structure logical? For example, do the sections appear in a logical order? Does the beginning of the article sufficiently orient readers to the scope and structure of the review? Are subheadings used effectively to make the structure apparent? If more than one level of subheading is used, does the hierarchy of topics appear appropriate?
- Is each section logically organized? For example, does each section begin with an overview, to orient readers and to serve skimmers who read just the beginnings of the sections? Does the flow of information in each section make sense? For example, depending on the subject matter, is the content presented chronologically, from most to least important, from head to toe, or in some other logical order?
- Are the paragraphs well structured? In particular, does each begin with a topic sentence that orients readers by stating the paragraph's subject and, if feasible, also serves skimmers by stating the paragraph's main point? Is the information in the body of each paragraph logically organized? Are transitions used well to help show the flow of ideas?
- Within paragraphs and at higher levels, is information from various sources well integrated? Review-article drafts by early-career authors sometimes just summarize each study in a paragraph of its own; thus, they resemble little more than a series of abstracts. A well-integrated review article not only presents key information about and from key studies but also shows how the different studies and their findings

relate to each other. For example, if relevant, they may show how successive studies extended knowledge, identify similarities and differences of findings of different studies, consider possible reasons for the differences, and, importantly, identify research gaps and recommend research to address them. Substantive editing can include assessing how well such items are done and identifying additional points at which such items might be worth doing.

- If tables, figures, or both are included, does each one contribute sufficiently to the review article to be worth retaining? Are figures and tables that seem worth retaining well designed? Might any tables or figures be worth adding, either to replace text or to supplement it?
- If conclusions are drawn, are they clearly supported by the evidence presented? If not: Should the reasoning behind the conclusions be made more explicit? Should the conclusions be stated less assertively? Should exceptions be noted? Or do other revisions seem advisable?

Such questions also may aid in substantively editing book chapters.

Editing a review article in the IMRAD format has much in common with editing a scientific paper in this format. Thus, much of the advice earlier in this chapter on editing IMRAD-structured articles applies. More specifically, in substantively editing an IMRAD-style review article, questions to address may include the following: Does the introduction make the focus of the review article clear? In particular, is it apparent what question(s) the review addressed? Are the methods of searching and analyzing the literature adequately documented? Are the findings presented in an appropriate amount of detail? And are they presented effectively? For example, if a table comparing the various studies would be useful, is one provided? If it is provided, is it well designed? And do the conclusions follow logically from the findings?

Much more guidance on editing systematic reviews and some other types of review articles can be gleaned from standardized guidelines for writing the respective article types. Such guidelines will be discussed later in this chapter.

CASE REPORTS

Case reports—in other words, articles describing and discussing noteworthy medical cases—can be useful additions to the medical literature.

Sometimes they add important new medical knowledge. For example, some describe newly recognized diseases; the literature on AIDS and that on COVID-19 began with case reports. Sometimes they report a previously unreported sign or symptom of a known disease, a newly recognized effect (favorable or unfavorable) of a drug, or other new knowledge relating to a case. Some other case reports do not present new knowledge but have educational value, for instance because they instruct or remind readers about proper diagnosis or treatment.

Normally, in human medicine, a case report may be published only if the patient has granted written permission. If the patient is too young to do so, is deceased, or is otherwise incapable of such actions, permission may be granted by a parent or guardian, the next of kin, or another appropriate person. Veterinary case reports should be published only with written permission of the animal's owner or another responsible party. An editor's role can include checking that the needed permission has been obtained.

A classically structured case report consists of an introduction, a case description, a discussion, and references. Commonly, there is also an abstract briefly summarizing the report. The *introduction* should provide context and say why the case is being reported. Normally, introductions to case reports are brief; thus, substantively editing them can include suggesting how to streamline them. Substantively editing the introduction also can include assessing its suitability for the audience. For example, the introduction to a case report in a general medical journal may need to include basic background; one in a journal for specialists will need less context. Also consider whether the introduction seems logically structured—for example progressing from general to specific, as in the introduction to a journal article reporting research. Finally, ensure that the introduction makes clear, typically at the end, why the case is being reported.

The *case description* usually presents information in a standard order: first the reason that medical attention was sought (sometimes called the "chief complaint"), then relevant points from the medical history and physical examination, then results of laboratory tests and other studies (such as imaging), then treatment, and then follow-up. Substantive editing includes ensuring that this order is followed throughout unless reasons exist to deviate and making sure that each part of the case description appears logically structured. It also entails, insofar as the substantive editor's background permits, checking whether all the needed information is present and identifying tangential information to consider deleting.

A substantive editor should make sure that the patient's identity is thoroughly concealed (except in the rare instances that the patient requests otherwise—as sometimes occurs when, for example, physicians publish case reports on their own illnesses). Deleting the patient's name or initials may not suffice. For example, if demographic information such as age (rather than age range), race or ethnicity, and occupation are not relevant medically, they should be omitted; especially in combination with information on the authors' affiliations (from which the patient's geographic location can often be inferred), such a combination of details may allow the patient's identity to be guessed. Similarly, even if a photograph does not include the patient's face, inclusion of a feature such as a distinctive tattoo may disclose the patient's identity; in such an instance, an editor may advise cropping the photo to remove the detail or, if doing so is impossible, not using the photograph.

The *discussion* section of a case report should be well focused, relating explicitly to the reason the case was reported. Questions to consider when substantively editing the discussion include the following:

- Has the case been related adequately to previous literature? For example, if somewhat similar cases have been reported, are sufficient comparisons made?
- If there are gaps or discrepancies in the report, are they addressed? For example, if a laboratory test that might have helped support the conclusion could not be obtained, or if results of some tests support a given conclusion but results of another test do not, do the authors discuss the implications?
- If relevant, are recommendations made? Are such recommendations sufficiently supported by the evidence from the case?

If answers to any such questions are "no," substantive editing may include suggesting further development of that aspect of the discussion. A substantive editor should also check whether the discussion appears logically structured. Like that of an article reporting research, the discussion section of a case report usually should move from specific to general. In this instance, doing so typically entails focusing first on the case, then placing it in the context of the literature, and ending with lessons learned from the case.

The reference lists of classically structured case reports usually are short. Often, they need only copyediting. However, if it seems that insufficient literature has been cited, that some cited works might not be credible sources, or that excessively many works have been cited, a substantive editor may be of service by raising the possibility with the authors.

Instead of the classic case report structure, some case reports follow the IMRAD format (introduction, methods, results, and discussion) or a variant of it. This format can serve especially well if evaluating the patient's condition included extensive laboratory investigations that would best be described in a methods section. In some regards, substantively editing an IMRAD-style case report resembles substantively editing an IMRAD-style research article; in other regards, it resembles editing a classic case report. Therefore, if you have an IMRAD-style case report to edit, you may find it useful to consult the parts of this chapter on each section.

Using Guidelines for Journal Article Types

Largely starting in the 1990s, standardized guidelines have been developed for the content and structure of journal articles reporting specific types of medical research, such as randomized clinical trials, and for other types of medical journal articles. These guidelines—often developed by groups including researchers and editors—help ensure that content is complete and effectively presented. The guidelines ease the work of authors by guiding them on what types of information to present and how to do so. They also assist substantive editors by serving essentially as checklists regarding content and structure. In addition, they aid readers by helping ensure that advisable content is present and by promoting use of standardized structures, which facilitate finding information being sought.

These guidelines are indeed guidelines, not laws. Some journals require using some of them, others not. Also, authors and editors should employ judgment in using them, for not every aspect is relevant in every instance, and sometimes items not specified are important to report. Nevertheless, awareness of these guidelines can aid considerably in substantive editing.

Some of the more general such guidelines have been published simultaneously in several journals, to publicize them and facilitate access. Also, more than 600 of the sets of guidelines can be accessed through the website of the EQUATOR (short for **E**nhancing the **QUA**lity and **T**ransparency **O**f health **R**esearch) Network (https://www.equator

-network.org/). (Those naming the website, and those naming many of the sets of guidelines, show a penchant for coining acronyms.)

Among the guidelines likely to be most broadly useful for substantive editing in medicine are the CONSORT guidelines (for reports of randomized clinical trials), the PRISMA guidelines (for systematic review articles), and the CARE guidelines (for case reports). Some details:

- The CONSORT (**CON**solidated **S**tandards **O**f **R**eporting **T**rials) statement was first issued in 1996 and has since been revised; links to current versions in several journals appear at https://www.equator-network.org/reporting-guidelines/consort/. One key feature is a 30-item checklist of items to include in respective sections of a scientific paper reporting a randomized, controlled trial. Another key feature is a standardized flow diagram to show how many individuals were assessed for eligibility, how many entered the trial, how many were randomized to each intervention, and so forth. Also listed on the EQUATOR website are specialized versions of the CONSORT statement—for example for clinical trials occurring in specific fields (such as orthodontia), involving specific categories of interventions, or employing particular types of designs.
- Current copies of the PRISMA (**P**referred **R**eporting **I**tems for **S**ystematic reviews and **M**eta-**A**nalyses) statement can be accessed at https://www.equator-network.org/reporting-guidelines/prisma/. PRISMA includes a checklist of content to provide. Most items in the checklist regard the methods and results sections. PRISMA also includes a checklist for the abstract and a standardized flow diagram for showing how the literature to include was narrowed down. The PRISMA entry on the EQUATOR website lists articles elaborating on the PRISMA statement or providing guidance on its use in specific contexts.
- The CARE (for **CA**se **RE**port) guidelines (see https://www.equator-network.org/reporting-guidelines/care/), like the CONSORT and PRISMA guidelines, include a largely section-by-section checklist of information to include. An associated article (Riley, Barber, Kienle, et al. 2017) offers elaboration, including examples of providing the types of information requested. For instance, the guidelines recommend including a timeline, and the article contains an example of such a timeline.

Among the many other guidelines accessible through the EQUATOR website are the STROBE (**ST**rengthening the **R**eporting of **OB**servational studies in **E**pidemiology) statement, which provides guidance in reporting cohort, case-control, and cross-sectional studies; the ARRIVE (**A**nimal **R**esearch: **R**eporting of **I**n **V**ivo **E**xperiments) guidelines, for reporting laboratory animal research; and the SRQR (**S**tandards for **R**eporting **Q**ualitative **R**esearch) guidelines. The EQUATOR website also allows searching by study type, clinical area, and section of report, as well as searching with free text. For example, a free-text search using the term "medical education" yields links to several sets of guidelines for literature in this regard.

Of course, such guidelines are primarily for authors, not editors. Many medical authors, though, are unaware that such guidelines exist. In such instances, editors can help by introducing the guidelines relevant to the authors' work. Doing so can both ease the authors' writing task and facilitate the substantive editing that follows.

Editing Medical Articles for General Readerships

In addition to editing journal articles, medical editing can include editing journalistic writing for general readerships. The latter includes news stories reporting findings of new medical research. It also includes news releases intended largely to obtain such coverage. And it includes feature stories. Pointers on editing these types of writing follow.

NEWS STORIES AND NEWS RELEASES

News stories on medical research appear in newspapers and magazines, in the broadcast media, on news websites, and elsewhere. They can be by staff or freelance journalists; sometimes the journalists have a background in medical writing or science writing, sometimes not. The stories tend to regard research on medical topics of broad public interest, such as common serious diseases. They tend to be written when an event makes them timely (in other words, when a "news peg" exists)—for example, when the research is presented at a conference or especially when a scientific paper reporting the research appears in a journal.

News releases (also known as *press releases*) resemble news stories but are intended to promote the research and the entity issuing the release.

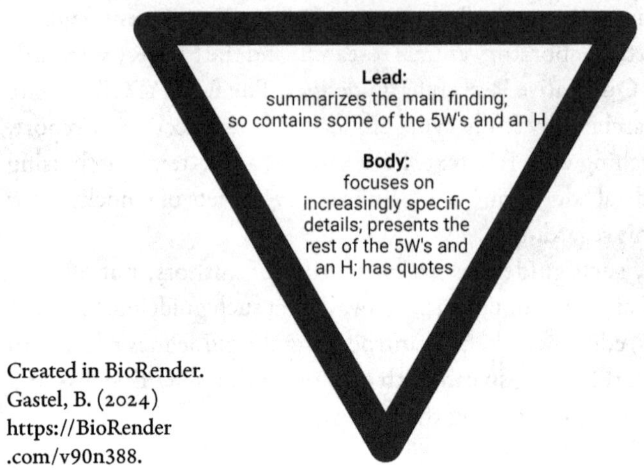

Created in BioRender.
Gastel, B. (2024)
https://BioRender
.com/v90n388.

They may be issued by the institution where the researchers work, the funder of the research, the journal publishing the research, or other entities associated with the research or its publication. They typically appear around the time the research is published. News releases are issued largely in the hope of obtaining coverage in the popular media. Thus, they are distributed to journalists, and sometimes they are posted on sites, such as EurekAlert! (https://www.eurekalert.org/), that journalists consult in search of story ideas. Journalists can then use the releases as starting points for writing about the research, and some media publish or post the releases as is. In addition, the entities issuing the news releases commonly post them on their own websites. Sometimes these entities also include the news releases or versions of them in their own media, such as internal newsletters or alumni magazines.

News stories generally are written in *inverted pyramid format*. In this format, the main point appears at the beginning, in what sometimes is called a *summary lead*. Progressively finer details follow. Thus, readers can grasp the key idea even if they do not finish the story—and sites publishing or posting the story can truncate it at any point (for instance, to meet space constraints) and still have it make sense. In the United States, news stories typically appear in AP (Associated Press) style; a major difference from AMA (American Medical Association) style is that the serial comma is rarely used. Typically in news stories, paragraphs are short, and quotations appear in paragraphs separate from other text. News releases generally employ the same style and format as news stories, in part so users wishing to do so can publish or post them as is.

A basic question for editors commissioning medical news stories or medical news releases is whether a given study is suited for coverage. Some medical research, though scientifically valuable, is too technical or specialized to be of broad public interest. And some research may be too preliminary for responsible coverage. For example, potential drugs require many years of testing in the laboratory, in animals, and then in humans to determine whether they are safe and effective and so can become available for use. And relatively few candidates pan out. Therefore, to avoid raising false or premature hopes, some media outlets avoid reporting on studies indicating that in animals—or test tubes—a potential drug shows promise.

Once a medical news story or medical news release is written, editing the two have much in common but also pose some different considerations. Questions to address in editing both include the following:

- Does the story include the journalistic five W's and an H (who, what, where, when, why, and how)? For example, does it say who did the research, what the research showed, where the research was done, where it was presented or published, when it was presented or published, why it is important, and how the research was done?
- Does the opening make the main point clear right away? (Some writers, especially early in their careers, present too much background information first. In inverted pyramid style, the background comes later.)
- Does the story or release also follow newswriting style in other regards? For example, are paragraphs fairly short, or should some be divided? Are quotes from people included, and, ideally, does a quote appear fairly early in the story?
- Is the piece medically accurate? Is the content consistent with that of the journal article, conference presentation, or other material on which the piece is based? Does the other medical information, such as that provided as background, appear correct?
- Is the piece suitable for a general readership? For example: Are technical terms avoided or defined? Is the reading level basic

enough? Is sufficient context included to understand the significance of the work? Are methodological details, which tend to interest few readers, either presented late in the story or avoided?

Because news releases have a promotional function, editing them also includes considerations in that regard. For example, the editor should ensure that the entity issuing the release (for example, the researchers' institution) is mentioned early in the release and, ideally, that one of the authors who is from the institution is quoted fairly early. The editor also should make sure that contact information—of one or more of the researchers, a *public information officer*, or both—is provided in case journalists want to follow up with interviews. And they should make sure that findings or implications are not overstated in a misguided attempt to advance the institution.

Whereas substantively editing a medical news release includes helping ensure sufficient focus on the issuing institution, substantively editing a medical news story includes helping ensure broad enough perspective. For instance: Does the story place the research in the context of earlier research? Have experts who were not involved (and who are not at the researchers' institution) commented on the research? Does the story mention limitations of the research? If the research indicates that an intervention (such as a diagnostic test, preventive measure, or treatment) is effective, how does it compare with other interventions for the same purpose? What about side effects or risks? Also, how much does the intervention cost? Does insurance currently cover the cost? And speaking of money, who funded the research? Do there seem to be conflicts of interest? Substantively editing a medical news story should attend to such considerations. And ideally, if the writer is not experienced, an editor should guide the writer along the way to make sure such considerations are addressed.

Another consideration regards review of a draft by people whose research is being reported or who are quoted. For stories for the media, the norm is not to allow such review, lest it lead to attempts to change the spin of the story. However, for such stories it can be acceptable for reporters to read people's quotes back to them, to check accuracy of the technical content. In contrast, for news releases, typical practice is to include review by the researchers. It can be helpful, though, to emphasize to the researchers that the review is for scientific accuracy, not style, and that the release has been written to serve general readers, not scientific peers. Some researchers request changes unsuitable for a news release—such as restoring technical language, listing many collaborators early in the release, or adding a lengthy description of research methods. In such situations, an editor may work with the writer and the researcher to come up with a version with which all parties are comfortable.

Another difference between news stories and news releases regards editing of quotes. For news stories, quotes must remain as uttered. At the most, the reporter or editor can correct grammar and delete fillers such as *um*, *er*, and *you know*. However, in institutional writing such as news releases, editing quotes more extensively tends to be permissible. For example, as long as the quoted person approves the edited version, the writer or editor may edit quotes for clarity, conciseness, or impact. Similarly, when reviewing drafts of news releases, those quoted may propose revisions of their quotes.

For both news stories and news releases, substantive editing can include guiding writers on choosing quotes or, if some quotes seem weak, suggesting that they be replaced or deleted. In general, quotes should not merely state information, especially if the writer could state it better. Rather, good quotes add insights, express opinions, show emotion, present ideas in fresh ways (for example, through lively wording or apt analogies), or otherwise contribute personality and perspective. Additional aspects of substantive editing of news stories or news releases can include evaluating or adding visual, audio, or video materials; providing or checking links to related items, such as the journal article reporting the research; and, for some venues such as EurekAlert!, providing or revising keywords.

FEATURE ARTICLES

In addition to news stories and news releases, publications and institutions often produce *feature articles* (also known as *feature stories*) on medical topics. Less time sensitive than news pieces, and often longer, they can focus on various types of topic. For example, they may profile a health professional, researcher, patient, or other person; explore a trend or development in medical research or medical care; offer health-related guidance; consider an issue in public health or medical ethics; recount, in lay terms, a mysterious medical case and its solution; or have any of myriad other emphases. Rather than being limited to inverted pyramid format, feature articles can have a range of structures, including chronological and subtopic-by-subtopic. Feature articles also may make use of literary devices such as similes, metaphors, and wordplay.

Editing feature articles includes many of the same aspects as editing news stories and news releases. For example, it includes ensuring that the reading level and technical level seem suitable for the intended readers; checking or querying content that seems likely to be incorrect; assessing quotes; and evaluating components other than text. It also includes other items. Among other aspects to address in substantively editing feature articles are the following dozen:

1. Is the beginning of the article (the *lead*, sometimes spelled *lede*) engaging and thus likely to make readers want to continue? If not, how could it be made more enticing?
2. If the lead does not indicate the focus and scope of the article, is it followed by a *nut graf* (also called a *billboard paragraph*) that does so? For instance, if the lead of an article on progress treating a disease depicts a patient's experience, the nut graf may say "Eddie Editor is one of eight zillion Americans with ampersand-asterisk disease. Living with this disease can pose frustrating challenges. But recent advances in treatment are minimizing its interference with patients' lives."
3. Is the article structured logically? Does it flow well? If not, how could structure or flow be improved?
4. If the article does not have subheadings, should some be added? If it has subheadings, are they sufficiently informative and engaging, and are the number and placement suitable?
5. Does the article contain sufficient human interest, such as stories of or quotes from health professionals, researchers, or patients? Are the humans appropriately diverse? For example: Are people of suitably varied ages, genders, races, and ethnicities represented? Whereas physicians have tended to be the only health professionals quoted, are there quotes from various types of health professionals with relevant expertise?
6. If people with a disease are portrayed, does the choice of people convey an accurate impression of the disease? For example, has the author resisted the temptation to present only the most severe cases or most successful treatment outcomes? Are hype and melodrama avoided?
7. Does the article seem to have a suitable tone throughout? For

example, levity may suit an article on hiccups, freckles, or flatulence. It is unlikely to suit an article on a terminal disease.

8. Does the article appear well paced? Or do parts seem likely to bog readers down—for example, because several difficult points are presented close together or a long stretch of text provides only dry information? If so, how could the pacing be improved? For example: Could each difficult point be followed by an example or a comment? Could the long dry passage be enlivened by quotes or anecdotes, or could parts be moved or deleted?
9. Does the article address the questions likely to come to mind as people read the article? Or do there seem to be unanswered questions? If so, where and how could they be addressed?
10. Does the article deliver what the lead or nut graf promised? If not, how would the discrepancy best be resolved? Would it be better to recast the lead or nut graf or to adjust the substance of the body of the article?
11. Does the article end well? Whereas a news story with an inverted pyramid structure can rightly fade into increasingly minor details, a feature generally should end strongly. For example, it might emphasize the message for readers to take away. Or it might circle back to the opening image, providing a satisfying closure. The ends and beginnings of the article, and of sections of the article, tend to attract particular attention. Try to ensure that the article takes advantage of this fact.
12. If appropriate, are sources of further information identified for readers wanting to know more?

For some feature articles, substantive editing also includes addressing visual or audiovisual aspects. For example, if graphics, audio, or video accompany the article, are they appropriate and of high quality? Would any such elements be worth adding? If visuals are presented, should captions be added or revised? Attention to such aspects can help a feature article excel in substance and style.

In short, substantive editing can help ensure that news stories, news releases, and feature articles contain suitable medically related content and communicate it well. Substantive editing following many of the same guidelines also can improve other types of journalistic medical writing, such as editorials and medical advice columns. Similarly, substantive editing can strengthen other types of writing that regard medicine or take place in medical contexts. The next section addresses an instance in this regard.

Editing Grant Proposals

Editing *grant proposals* (also known as *grant applications*) that seek funding for biomedical research is sometimes a specialty in itself. Some health science centers and other institutions hosting considerable biomedical research have one or more editors who specialize in editing grant applications. Some freelance medical editors also focus at least largely on this realm. Given the different requirements of different funders, the varied categories of grants from funding sources such as the US National Institutes of Health, and the complexity of some types of grant applications, editing biomedical grant proposals can itself be the subject of a substantial book. Nevertheless, even a general medical editor can do much to strengthen a grant proposal and thus increase its likelihood of funding. To help ensure that a proposal is clear, readable, and persuasive, such editing typically includes a mix of copyediting and substantive editing.

Requirements regarding the structure and length of grant proposals differ among funding sources and sometimes among grant categories from the same funding source. However, most grant proposals have the following elements in common: a title; an abstract (or another type of section summarizing the proposal); a section presenting background information; a statement of aims, objectives, hypotheses, or research questions; a research plan (or a project plan if, for example, the grant would be for an educational program or service program); information about qualifications of the project team; and a budget. Editing may strengthen all these components.

Funders commonly require biomedical research grant proposals to have a section known as *specific aims*. This section, typically limited to one page, concisely justifies the proposed research, provides context, identifies the hypotheses to be tested, and says how they will be tested. The specific aims section tends to be the core of the proposal. Other sections elaborate on it, and, as it serves as a brief and readily identifiable summary, peer reviewers pay particular attention to it. In editing a proposal, it can be advisable to focus on the specific aims section early on, to ascertain the essence of the proposed research. Returning periodically to this section also can be prudent, to help ensure that it and other sections are consistent. If a draft of a grant proposal arrives too late to permit thorough editing of the entire proposal, it can be wise to concentrate largely on editing the specific aims section, given its importance.

A grant proposal is a type of persuasive writing. It must persuade the funding source (or the peer reviewers that advise it) that the proposed work is consistent with the funding source's priorities and that the work will be done excellently. Sources of biomedical funding generally receive many more proposals for good research than they can fund. Thus, to be funded, a proposal must show that the work will be especially relevant and outstanding. Failure to be persuasive in one or more regards may be grounds for the funder or reviewers to rate a proposal too low to fund, or to suggest that the proposal be strengthened and then resubmitted the next time around. Among questions a substantive editor may consider in trying to ensure that a proposal is persuasive are the following:

- Is the goal clearly worthwhile? For example, if the research will regard a given disease, does the proposal contain statistics demonstrating the disease's importance?
- Does the goal clearly match the funder's mission? For example, if the funder's mission regards a given disease but the proposal is for research in basic science, does the proposal explicitly state how the basic science relates to the disease?
- Do the methods suit the goal? For example, does the proposal make explicit how the stated methods would help test the hypothesis?
- Are the personnel clearly qualified? For example, if the research will require use of an advanced technique, is it clear from the proposal that a team member will have the needed expertise with that technique?
- Are the facilities clearly adequate? For example, if specialized laboratory facilities will be needed, is it clear from the proposal that those facilities are available?
- Is the budget clearly appropriate? For instance, do all the listed materials correspond to tasks described in the proposal? If people are to be paid, does the payment seem commensurate with the work?

If a proposal seems less than persuasive in any such regards, substantive editing may include pointing out to the author the areas that would seem likely to benefit from strengthening—and, ideally, pointing out potential ways to strengthen them.

Some examples of other questions to consider are as follows:

- Have all instructions been followed? Some funding sources have stringent instructions regarding the content and format of proposals; failure to follow the instructions may disqualify a proposal. Therefore, checking for compliance with the instructions can be an important service.
- Is the proposal at a suitable level? For funding agencies such as the US National Institutes of Health, researchers in the same field as those submitting the proposals evaluate the proposals. Therefore, the proposals can be fairly technical. For some other funding sources, such as community-based foundations, the reviewers sometimes include laypeople interested in the funder's mission. In that case, the proposal should be written such that educated members of the general public can understand it. Usually, the researcher writing the proposal knows, or can find out, what types of people will review the proposal. The researcher can then inform the editor so that, if warranted, the technical level of the proposal can be adjusted.
- Does the proposal flow well? Proposal reviewers tend to be very busy and to have many proposals to evaluate. Therefore, they cannot be expected to invest the time and effort needed to intuit connections between ideas in a proposal. Rather, the proposal should make the relationships of the ideas apparent. Good organization can aid greatly in this regard. So can appropriate use of transitional words and phrases.
- Is the proposal consistent throughout? As a proposal is written and revised, inconsistencies may develop. The author might correct some data in a table but neglect to do so in the corresponding text. Or the author might revise the number of animals to study but forget to update the budget accordingly. Likewise, an editor might make a change in format but not apply it consistently. Inconsistencies, especially in content, can confuse reviewers and undermine the credibility of a proposal. Therefore, checking for consistency can be an important part of editing a proposal.
- If warranted, are tables and figures used? For instance, if a research proposal contains preliminary findings (as is often advisable), tables and figures can aid in their presentation. Or if a proposal is for a service project, a timeline can clarify the plans and help show

that they are well conceived and feasible. Of course, any tables and figures should be designed for clarity. To help ensure that a proposal communicates well, consider whether any tables or figures should be added, deleted, or revised.

- Is the proposal readably written and easy to skim? Reviewers of proposals tend to be chosen in part because of their prominence and productivity. Thus, they usually are very busy and may be tired and harried. (Envision a reviewer who has spent a long day addressing lab issues, teaching students, attending meetings, and perhaps caring for patients; who has dealt with household duties for much of the evening; and who finally, late at night, has multiple proposals to review.) To help the reviewer accurately grasp the proposal's content—and to prevent the reviewer's assessment from being clouded by frustration at trying to ascertain what the author was trying to say—make the proposal easy to read and skim. For example, perhaps add subheadings to guide readers, use italics or boldface to call attention to key points, and break long, convoluted sentences into more than one sentence apiece. Further guidance in this regard appears in the section "Editing for Readability" in chapter 7.

Problems common in grant proposals include excessive use of abbreviations (including especially acronyms) and failure to define the abbreviations. To avoid confusion, abbreviations in a proposal should be limited largely to those that are standard and already familiar to reviewers. Normally, each abbreviation should be defined the first time it appears. And usually, an abbreviation should be used only if the term will appear more than a few times; otherwise, the risk of confusion outweighs the space saved. If a proposal uses multiple abbreviations that might be unfamiliar to some reviewers, adding a table of abbreviations can help. Also, if a proposal is lengthy, it can be worthwhile to define an abbreviation the first time it appears in any given section, especially if the sections might not always be read consecutively.

Like journal articles, grant proposals cite references and include reference lists. Thus, substantive editing of a grant proposal includes helping to ensure that references are cited when needed and that the reference list is up-to-date and is otherwise thorough yet focused. If reviewing the literature more thoroughly seems likely to benefit the proposal, perhaps suggest that the authors consult a research librarian at their institution.

Grants usually should lead to journal articles reporting the results of the funded work. In substantively editing a grant proposal, it can be helpful to consider whether the work as proposed would yield all the information needed for this purpose. If research is being proposed, would it produce all the data required? If education or service is being proposed, would the project include sufficient evaluation to be readily publishable? Sometimes proposal authors and editors envision tables and figures that would appear in resulting papers and check whether the work would yield all the data needed to complete them. Working backward in this way can identify gaps to fill in a proposal.

Some funders have two-stage processes for proposal submission. First, applicants submit brief preliminary proposals summarizing what they wish to propose. These preliminary proposals are evaluated, and the applicants with the strongest ones are invited to submit full proposals. The full proposals are then reviewed for potential funding. Editors may edit both preliminary and final proposals. Editing preliminary proposals can be especially valuable, as they must be convincing so the applicants can reach the next stage but also must be highly concise.

Preparing a proposal for a large grant—which may total hundreds of thousands of dollars—is an extensive endeavor, often taking six months or more. It typically involves multiple people, including the main person proposing the project (the *principal investigator*), others slated for major roles in it, and support staff. If possible, an editor should become involved early in the planning stage, when content and organization are being decided and therefore large-scale substantive suggestions can best be provided. An editor may also help develop a timeline for writing and editing the parts of the proposal. More broadly, sometimes the editor assumes a project management role—for example, ensuring that contributors submit their components on time, gathering curricula vitae or biosketches of team members, assembling letters of support from administrators and outside collaborators, and the like. If different people write different parts of the proposal, the editor generally should edit the parts for consistency (or at least compatibility) of style. An editor can contribute much to helping a grant proposal achieve its potential.

Finally, a word on wording: People often speak of "writing a grant" or "editing a grant." However, the grant is the funding, not the request for it. Sometimes when people say "I'm writing a grant," I'm tempted to respond, "While you have your checkbook out, please write one for me." Formally speaking, unless you are a funder, the proper wording is "writing (or editing) a grant proposal" or "writing (or editing) a grant application."

Key Points

- Substantive editing addresses largely content and organization. It therefore can help ensure the validity of medical writing. It also can increase the impact of such writing.
- Aspects to address in substantive editing include completeness, focus, organization, logic, and ethics.
- Journal articles reporting medical research usually follow the IMRAD format: introduction, methods, results, and discussion. They thus have an hourglass structure, moving from broad context, to narrow focus on the research being reported, back to broad context. Substantive editing of an IMRAD article includes editing for compliance with this structure.
- Medical editing also includes editing other types of journal articles, such as review articles and case reports. Each of these two can have either a traditional narrative-like structure or an IMRAD-like structure. The editing should be in keeping with the structure used.
- Guidelines exist for specific journal article types, such as clinical-trial reports, systematic review articles, and case reports. Many of these guidelines can be accessed through the EQUATOR website. The guidelines can aid both authors and editors.
- In editing medical articles for general readerships, journalistic conventions should be followed. These conventions include use of the inverted pyramid structure for news articles and news releases.
- Editing grant proposals can increase their clarity, credibility, and persuasiveness. Thus, it can increase their likelihood of acceptance. Ideally, a substantive editor should be involved starting early in the proposal preparation process.

· EXERCISE ·
Organization of a Journal Article

Substantive editors of journal articles reporting medical research must assess whether statements are in the correct section. Please write I, M, R, or D after each sentence to indicate whether it is likely to fit best in the introduction, methods section, results section, or discussion.

1. The objective of our study was to determine whether Procedure A is superior to Procedure B.
2. Whole-genome sequencing was performed with the use of Illumina MiSeq.
3. All deaths were classified by using the International Classification of Diseases, 11th Revision.
4. Future studies should quantify the magnitude of this type of activity.
5. Of the 3478 screening swabs, 183 (5.3%) yielded one or more isolates.
6. _____ is an emerging pathogen that has recently been associated with outbreaks worldwide.
7. Participants aged 25 to 50 years who were referred to 1 of 6 participating hospitals were eligible for inclusion.
8. Our findings are consistent with the pooled results of earlier trials.
9. In total, 120 (40%) of the 300 nurses responded to questions in the survey.
10. Our current study has several limitations.
11. RNA was isolated by Hinton method II (39).
12. Our results indicate that reusable patient equipment may serve as a source of health care-associated outbreaks of infection with this agent.
13. We emailed the survey to 375 academic authors in September 2024.
14. Figure 3 shows the changes in function during the 2-year follow-up period.
15. The findings of our current study add to the body of research showing an association between ____ and ____.
16. Twelve dogs in the XYZ group and 11 dogs in the control group had complete healing at the 2-week reevaluation.
17. The Student *t* test was used to identify differences between groups.
18. The healing rate resembled that in a previous study of this intervention.
19. Significantly lower rates were found in patients with ABC ($P = .024$).
20. Our hypothesis was that ___ may predispose patients with XYZ to develop cancer.
21. This finding is in complete contrast to our expectation.
22. Patients were stratified by sex and by ethnic group.

23. Another possible explanation for this finding may be related to continuous treatment with ______.
24. After autoradiography, films were scanned using a Powerlook 100XL densitometer (Bio-Rad).
25. These findings are especially interesting in the context of HIV vaccine development.

· EXERCISE ·

Providing Substantive Feedback on an Abstract

Imagine that an author gives you the draft below. It is an early draft, and so the author is seeking feedback mainly on content and organization. (1) List current strengths of the draft. (2) Suggest improvements. The sentences are numbered to aid in doing so. Your feedback should be worded such that a message to the author could include it.

Comparison of Methods to Help Authors Submit Better Abstracts

Background. [1]Medical journals receive many papers with poorly written abstracts. [2]According to recent studies (Gwosdow 2023; Duncan and Murphy 2024), the abstracts of more than 70% of submitted papers have major problems in content or crafting. [3]Therefore, the authors undertook a study of ways to improve abstracts accompanying papers that are submitted to medical journals.

Methods. [4]Researchers at major medical centers were assigned to attend a lecture on writing abstracts for journal articles, complete an online training module on this subject, receive daily time to take a nap, or receive no intervention. [5]The abstracts of the first papers they then submitted to journals were evaluated using the GOKW rubric. [6]The journal editors also were asked to rate the abstracts. [7]Statistical procedures such as chi-square tests and *t* tests were used.

Results. [8]Participants receiving daily nap time scored significantly higher when compared to the other 3 groups (Table 2). [9]No other significant differences were observed. [10]In the interviews, however, participants completing the online module said they became more confident of their ability to write excellent abstracts. [11]Perhaps this was because of the beautiful graphical abstracts shown in the module.

Conclusions. [12]Researchers at major medical centers tend to be sleep-deprived. [13]Over 70% of those interviewed in this study said so. [14]Policies should be instituted to increase the amount and quality of sleep that such researchers receive. [15]This study was supported by a grant from the Rip Van Winkle Institute.

· 6 ·

Editing Conference and Career Communications

Although many medical editors focus on editing articles or grant proposals, medical editing also can include editing other items presenting medically related content. Such items can include conference communications such as oral presentations, poster presentations, and proceedings. They also can include materials such as nomination letters and application essays. Often, the editing entails both copyediting and substantive editing. The current chapter therefore provides guidance on editing conference communications and more. The approaches also can apply to editing medically related items not specifically addressed in this chapter or other chapters.

Editing Conference Communications: Presentations and More

Medically related conferences typically include oral presentations and poster presentations. Medical presentations also are given in other contexts, such as courses for students and health professionals, events for the public, and interviews for medical faculty positions. Sometimes prospective conference presenters must submit abstracts of their proposed presentations. Also, at institutions presenting conferences or other events, medical editors may edit the program and other materials. Sometimes conferences are followed by editing and publication of *proceedings*, consisting mainly of papers presented. Thus, conferences and other events are associated with a variety of communications that can benefit from editing. Guidance follows.

ABSTRACTS, ETC.

Typically, those wanting to present at a conference must submit abstracts of the research they wish to share. Committees then review the abstracts and decide which proposed presentations to accept. The abstracts resemble those for journal articles, but sometimes the instructions differ, for example regarding length or inclusion of visuals. An editor can facilitate acceptance of abstracts by helping to ensure that they follow the instructions and are informative, well organized, clear, and concise. Readability can be especially important, as committee members often must review many abstracts in a short time.

If an abstract is accepted, the presenter may have pre-conference writing tasks in addition to preparing the oral or poster presentation. Such tasks may include revising the abstract to suit it for the conference program and providing a brief bio. With these tasks too, an editor may help regarding both substance and style.

SLIDE PRESENTATIONS

Medical presentations at conferences and in other settings almost always include slides. Images in the slides can help attract and retain audience members' attention, clarify content, and aid information retention. Likewise, text in the slides can foster understanding and learning. But slides also can detract and distract—for example, if (as often occurs) the slides are too numerous for the available time, the slides are too crowded, or the images are not quickly understandable. The following are some items to check in editing slides to help them fulfill their function well.

General aspects: One general aspect to consider is the number of slides in the presentation. An overall guideline is to average about one slide per minute. If this guideline is greatly exceeded, perhaps recommend deleting some slides. Other general aspects to consider include whether the slides are at a suitable technical level for the audience; whether the presentation has a logical, effective organization; and whether the presentation is consistent and cohesive in design. Check also whether some slides seem crowded; if so, look into removing minor content or dividing the material into more than one slide. Also consider whether language barriers may exist. For instance, if many audience members may understand written better than spoken English (as is often true at international conferences) or if the presenter speaks English with a heavy accent, perhaps include more text on the slides than otherwise would be used. Also, if an audience will be multilingual, consider including text in more than one language or simultaneously projecting slides in a second language.

The images: Editing slides also includes assessing images and, if warranted, proposing revisions or alternatives. Images in slides should be designed for rapid understanding. Therefore, graphs generally are preferable to tables in this context. The graphs and other images should be relatively simple, for quick comprehension; accordingly, some images from websites, books, or journals may need simplification. Also, if an image comes from such a source, ensure that a credit line is included.

The text: Slides tend to be too wordy, and so editing their text usually entails streamlining it for easy reading. General guidelines include limiting the text to no more than about seven lines other than the title, using mainly type of at least 28 points (except for items such as credit lines, which can be much smaller), and using bulleted lists rather than paragraphs. For readability, bulleted items can be words or phrases rather than sentences; in a given list, though, either all items should be phrases or all should be sentences, and parallelism also should exist in other regards. Also ensure that the typeface is suitable. Whereas serif typefaces

---

Editing Slide Presentations: A Checklist

- Is the number of slides reasonable for the length of the presentation (typically, about one slide per minute)?
- Are the slides in a consistent format?
- For easy reading onscreen, is a sans serif typeface (such as Calibri) used?
- Is the text large enough (ideally, at least about 28 point for major items)?
- Are the slides sufficiently uncrowded? If not, should some content be deleted, or should the material be divided into more than one slide?
- Is text kept relatively brief, for example by using bulleted lists of phrases?
- For quick comprehension, are graphs rather than tables used where possible?
- Are figures kept relatively simple, for rapid understanding?
- If images aren't the speaker's own, are credit lines provided?
- Are visuals designed such that viewers with color perception difficulties can understand them?
- If people with visual disabilities might view the slides on a screen reader, is alt text describing the images included?

(such as Times New Roman) work well in manuscripts, they tend to look messy in slides; instead, a sans serif typeface (such as Calibri, Aptos, or Arial) should be used.

Accessibility to all: Finally, check for accessibility. Many people have trouble distinguishing colors, especially red and green. Therefore, comprehensibility should not depend solely on color. For example, if bars in a bar graph are different colors, they also should have different patterns; or if lines in a graph are different colors, the data points should have different shapes, or the lines should have different patterns (such as solid, dotted, and dashed). Also consider using or suggesting a color palette designed for accessibility to people with color perception difficulties; online searching can reveal various such palettes. If the slides will be distributed to attendees or others, the images should have *alt text*, so people who have visual problems and therefore use screen readers can find out what is shown; sources of guidance in composing and thus editing alt text include *The Open Notebook* (2024). Finally, in keeping with the other advice on editing slides, strive to keep them uncluttered. They will then support the speaker in communicating best to the most.

POSTER PRESENTATIONS

Medical and scientific conferences commonly include poster presentations. In such a presentation, the author summarizes a research project (or other project) on a large poster. Traditionally, the posters have been printed on paper. Sometimes they are printed on cloth, for ease of transportation. In recent years, there also have been electronic posters, which are projected rather than printed; some are static, like printed posters, and others are dynamic, with videos or interactive elements. Of course, at virtual conferences, the posters are electronic.

Conferences typically include poster sessions, at which the presenters accompany their posters and discuss them with attendees. Commonly, the posters also are on display during other parts of the conferences. After conferences, many speakers display their posters in or near their offices or laboratories.

Posters at conferences vary widely in quality. Some are visually appealing and readily comprehensible. Many others are not, most often because they are too crowded. An editor can help the author ensure that a poster communicates well and attracts viewers. For greatest effectiveness and efficiency, the presenter and editor should work together starting in the planning phase. However, even if given a near-final draft, an editor can suggest improvements that help a poster achieve its objectives.

In working with a presenter to plan a poster, of course make sure that all instructions from the conference organizer will be followed. Be especially attentive to the instructions regarding size; if a poster exceeds the stated dimensions, space might not be available to display it. Also consider the interests and technical level of the attendees. Emphasize that a poster can successfully convey only a limited amount of content, and thus that the topic should be narrow enough and only highlights should be presented. Note that posters are largely a visual medium and therefore, if feasible, they should revolve around images that present key messages and attract viewers. Also note that a poster should contain relatively little text—usually about 500 to 1000 words (the equivalent of two to four average-length abstracts, or two to four double-spaced pages of text). Indeed, a poster is essentially an illustrated extended abstract.

A poster presenting research generally should be organized like a scientific paper or abstract: with an introduction (or background) section, a methods section, a results section, and a discussion (or conclusions) sec-

Editing Poster Presentations: A Checklist

- Have all instructions (for example, regarding poster dimensions) been followed?
- Is the poster title large enough—typically at least 72 points (1 inch or 2.5 centimeters)? Is the title informative and engaging?
- Is the poster logically organized—for example, in the IMRAD (introduction, methods, results, and discussion) format?
- Does the poster have enough white space to be appealing and easy to follow?
- Are the typefaces well chosen (for example, a standard sans serif typeface for headings and a standard serif typeface for the main text)?
- Is the text sufficiently brief (typically no more than 500 to 1000 words total)?
- Is the body type large enough for easy reading (commonly about 24 points)?
- For readability, are bulleted lists rather than paragraphs used where feasible?
- Are images chosen that both attract and inform?
- Are the images of high quality?
- Are the images simple enough to understand quickly?
- Can the images be understood by people with color perception difficulties?
- Do the figures have captions and, if warranted, credit lines?
- Is color used effectively? For example: Is the color scheme appropriate and cohesive? If relevant, is color used to call attention to key items?
- Is the presenter's contact information included?
- Are the mechanics of the writing correct throughout?

tion. If a poster will be in landscape format, it generally should have three to five columns; if in portrait format, it generally should have at least two columns. Unless the instructions require an abstract to be included, the poster should not contain one; little point exists to using a quarter to half of the available word count for information that will be repeated.

Attendees' decision to view a poster depends largely on the title. Therefore, it deserves careful editorial attention. The title should be informative, and it should be short enough to be readily readable (typically, no more than one line of text). Witty titles are appreciated at some conferences but not others; if in doubt, a straightforward title is safer. The title should be large enough for people strolling through the session to read easily; a general guideline is for it to be at least about 1 inch (2.5 centimeters) high—or, in other words, in at least 72-point type. Unless required by the conference organizers, the title generally should not be in all capital letters. One reason is that capital letters differ less in size and shape than lowercase letters do, and so words in all capital letters are harder to read. Another reason is that capital letters are wider on average than lowercase ones and so take up more space.

In advising presenters about images to include in a poster, or in helping presenters to refine this aspect, keep the following points in mind. Ideally, the images in a poster should both attract and inform. Of course, the results section generally should include images, such as graphs and photos. Images also can strengthen the methods section; for example, a flowchart may portray a protocol more clearly and engagingly than text would. Where feasible, graphs—which are easier to understand quickly—should be used rather than tables. Both graphs and tables should be simple, and they should be large enough to view easily. Be sure that each image has a caption or label, so viewers will understand it even if the presenter is absent or is talking with other attendees. Also consider placement of images; for greatest impact, the most important images generally should appear in a middle column and slightly above the center of the poster.

Help make sure that the poster employs color effectively. Like other aspects of design, color should promote communication rather than distracting from it. Normally, a poster should have a cohesive color scheme rather than seemingly random use of colors. Using a color scheme related to the topic (for example, predominantly green for an environmental health subject) supports the theme. And using a color scheme associated with the presenter's institution or program assists in branding. Making the most important images most colorful attracts attention to them. Also, making items that are related to each other, such as icons or headings, the same color helps show that they are related. Color also can aid in differentiating items in a graph or diagram. Remember, though, that some attendees have difficulty in perceiving colors. Therefore, ensure that graphs and other content will be readily understandable even if viewers cannot distinguish the colors, for example by following suggestions in that regard from this chapter's section on oral presentations. Similarly, if a poster might be viewed with screen readers, alt text should be included.

In editing the text as well, strive to promote quick and easy comprehension. Because a poster should have relatively little text, edit vigorously for conciseness. Where feasible, convert material in paragraphs into bulleted or numbered lists. Where paragraphs are used, keep them short. Ensure that the type is large enough for viewers to read easily: commonly about 24 points. Also assess the choices of typeface; using a sans serif typeface for headings and a serif typeface for body text can promote easy reading. Make sure that the poster contains the presenter's contact information, in case those viewing the poster without the presenter wish to follow up. If the poster lists many references, suggest that the presenter use fewer, if any, in keeping with the norms for posters.

Also consider items to suggest adding if not present. One such item is a *QR code* that visitors can scan to access a copy of the poster or obtain further information about the presenter's work. Another is a "key findings" box in the results section.

Further guidance on editing poster presentations can be gleaned from resources on designing them. One excellent such resource is the webpage "Designing Conference Posters" (https://colinpurrington.com/tips/poster-design/). Also, extensive guidance appears in the book *Better Posters* (Faulkes 2021). This book grew out of the blog "Better Posters" (https://betterposters.substack.com/); some posts in this blog are poster critiques indicating edits that can improve poster presentations.

CONFERENCE PROCEEDINGS AND ANALOGOUS WORKS

Medical editors sometimes edit works that are collections of articles or chapters by different authors. Some of these works are conference proceedings, consisting of papers that authors have prepared for a conference; these proceedings may appear as books, as supplements to journals, or in freestanding online formats. Other such multiauthor works are textbooks, or other books, for which authors write chapters on different aspects of the subject. Typically, one or more specialists on the medical subject matter determine and oversee the content of the proceedings, textbook, or other work and so are listed as editors. The professional medical editor, as a manuscript editor, works to ensure that the writing is mechanically sound, readable, and in a consistent style and format. Sometimes the medical editor also performs substantive editing, helping to refine the content and organization. The medical editor also may have a managerial role—for example, reminding authors to submit their contributions and revisions on time and otherwise helping to manage the project.

Although medical editors' duties vary somewhat among such multiauthor projects, some general guidelines commonly apply. The following are some to consider.

Become involved early—and provide instructions early. The following situation is all too common:

> The content experts in charge of a proceedings or other multiauthor work have compiled contributions, which they then conclude could benefit from editing. Therefore, a medical editor is called in. The medical editor finds that the contributions vary widely in style and format, quality of writing, and other regards—and perhaps that some contributions have not yet been submitted. Later, the medical editor also finds that some authors did not expect to be asked for revisions.

Such situations can be largely avoided by involving the medical editor early. If you are approached about editing such a work—or if you see that you might be—try to become involved as early as possible, while the work still is being planned. Especially if your role will include substantive editing, take part in planning the content and organization; even if not, arrange if possible to be privy to such discussions, for context. In coordination with the organizers, prepare a concise set of instructions to authors, specifying items such as lengths of contributions, bibliographic format, and deadlines for initial submissions and any revisions. Accompany the instructions with a brief message introducing yourself and describing your role. Send these materials to the authors as early as possible, perhaps ideally with a cover note from the organizers. Alas, at least one author may well disregard what you send. But overall, this approach provides the foundation for efficient, minimally stressful editing later.

Include some give in the schedule. As implied by the previous item, work with the organizers to develop a timetable for the project. Include some give, as delays commonly occur: Almost invariably some authors are late; you yourself may fall behind, for any of a variety of reasons; and technical or other delays may arise. Include enough flexibility to be likely to be able to compensate.

If relevant, start coordinating early with the publisher. If the work will be a journal supplement or book, contact the journal or book publisher to ensure that instructions to authors are consistent and to coordinate schedules and roles. If the work will be self-published or self-posted, start attending to logistics.

Develop a style sheet. To help ensure consistency within and between contributions, between rounds of editing, and (if applicable) between individuals involved in the editing, develop a thorough style sheet. Of course, specify standard editorial items such as main style manual and dictionary used, conventions followed for items such as punctuation and number format, and formats for citations and references. In the alphabetical list of terms, include items specific to the project. Such items may include, for example, technical terms, names of people and institutions, and specialized abbreviations used. Depending on the nature of the project, the main style sheet may be supplemented by specialized style sheets for individual contributions.

If appropriate, incorporate one or more rounds of revision. Like other writing, contributions to such multiauthor works benefit from revision. Therefore, in consultation with the organizers, consider incorporating revision into the schedule. Possible sources of feedback for such revision include the organizers, the medical editor, external reviewers, or (quite likely) some combination. As medical editor, you may be responsible for coordinating the feedback from the various sources. If the contributions are for a conference proceedings, a round of revision before the conference can help the presentations achieve their potential.

If the work is a conference proceedings, attend the conference if feasible. Attending the conference can have multiple benefits. Hearing the presentations and discussion can provide helpful context for embarking on or finalizing the editing. Meeting the contributors at the conference can promote rapport with them and thus facilitate editing. Unresolved questions about a contribution sometimes are readily resolved by talking with the author at the conference. Also, an editor who has been working on the proceedings, and so already is well versed in the conference content, may be especially well suited for tasks such as drafting a conference summary and preparing reports on conference discussions.

For a conference proceedings, allow final revisions after the conference, if possible. Based on discussion at the conference, speakers may have points to add to their contributions or other modifications to make. Likewise, editors may have new insights that can improve their editing of some contributions. Therefore, even if the contributions have been edited beforehand, allowing time after the conference for revisions can be worthwhile. Normally, this time should be short, so as not to lose momentum and not to delay release of the proceedings.

Track work carefully (for example, by revision number). Editing a conference proceedings, multiauthor book, or analogous project generally entails keeping track of successive versions of multiple contributions. Therefore, careful tracking is important. Spreadsheets and project management software can, of course, help. Especially important is a system for naming files so as to clearly designate versions. For example, successive versions of a contribution might be labeled as follows: Tuda_original, Tuda_edit 01-20250116, Tuda_edit 01_rev by author, and Tuda_edit 02-20250214. Try to avoid file names that are so long as to be unwieldy.

If relevant, plan to edit front matter and back matter. As editor, you probably will be responsible for editing—and might be responsible for compiling—the table of contents. You may also be involved in compiling and editing other elements, such as contributor bios, lists of conference participants, and appendixes. Likewise, if the volume has an index, your role might include editing it.

If relevant, participate in reviewing proofs. Once the proceedings, textbook, or other work reaches the proof stage, you might be among those reviewing the proofs. In doing so, it can be helpful to consult the style sheet(s) that you prepared for the project. The proofreading guidance in the next chapter also may be useful.

Editing a conference proceedings or multiauthor book can be among the largest and most challenging projects of a medical editor. However, it can also be among the most satisfying. In the midst of all the editing and coordination, you might state that you will never accept such a project again. Yet after you see the final product emerge, you may be pleased to undertake another such editing project—at least after a brief respite.

Editing Career-Related Communications

Medical editors who work at institutions such as health-professional schools or who freelance sometimes edit writings intended to demonstrate people's qualifications. Such writings include recommendation letters, application essays, and curricula vitae or resumes. Substantive editing and copyediting can help ensure that such writings are persuasive, readable, and polished. The following are suggestions for editing such writings.

RECOMMENDATION, EVALUATION, AND NOMINATION LETTERS

Letters recommending applicants for admission or employment . . . Letters evaluating candidates for promotion . . . "Dean's letters" (officially termed Medical Student Performance Evaluations) for residency applicants . . . Letters nominating scientists, clinicians, students, and others for awards . . . And more. Many such letters are written in academic medicine and other medically related settings. And occasion often arises to edit them.

As in other substantive editing, initial items to check include compliance with requirements. Those to whom such letters are to be submitted often state requirements regarding content, length, organization, or other items. Lack of compliance can decrease a letter's chances of success or even disqualify it from consideration. More generally, substantive editing includes evaluating how well the letter's content corresponds to explicit or implicit criteria by which the candidate will be evaluated. Should any content be added in order to demonstrate better the person's level of qualification? On the other hand, is there content that seems tangential and so might best be deleted? Substantive editing of letters can well include querying about such items.

Substantive editing also includes seeing whether assertions are, if feasible, supported with evidence. If a letter says a biomedical scientist's research is impactful, does it say how much the scientist's papers have been cited and, if applicable, how the research has contributed to health? If a letter says a clinician is extraordinarily devoted to patients, are examples provided? If a letter describes a faculty member as an innovative medical teacher, are innovations described? If a letter says a student is exceptionally service-oriented, does it show how the student's service has exceeded norms? Suggesting such documentation, if not yet present, can substantially strengthen a letter.

Another item to check for is the technical level. Some such letters go to groups consisting of specialists in the same field as the person being written about; other such letters go to groups that include others. The letter writer or the editor often has information in this regard or can obtain it. The technical level can then be adjusted if needed. More broadly, an editor can help ensure that all content is likely to be clear to all readers. For example, if a letter refers to an event that is known only locally but the letter will go to national or international readers, the editor should suggest explaining what the event is (or should draft an explanation and query whether to use it).

Drafts of letters such as those recommending people for awards commonly exceed the stated page limits. Therefore, editing such letters often entails shortening them. Doing so tends to include both deleting low-priority content and condensing the remaining content (in keeping with guidance the next chapter presents on editing for conciseness). Revising a letter to meet space constraints sometimes also includes slight reformatting, such as using a different typeface or slightly adjusting the margins. Beware, however, of major reformatting; extreme measures such as using minuscule type or tiny margins may undermine the effectiveness of a letter.

Those of us substantively editing such letters usually copyedit them as well. If more than one draft will be edited, much of the copyediting can wait until a later draft, in which the content has been essentially finalized. Editing such letters for clarity and readability can be especially important because readers of such letters often are busy and tired and have many letters to review. Also, ensuring that the letter is mechanically sound—without errors in grammar, spelling, punctuation, or word use—helps ensure that the letter will appear credible, that it will make a good impression, and that readers will not be distracted by problems with the writing.

Final items to check include whether the letter begins and ends strongly. (Final checking of the beginning and end tends to best wait until late in the substantive editing because these items must be consistent with the rest of the letter.) Normally, the opening paragraph should identify the person being written about, say what the person is being considered for, and indicate the overall message of the letter. Also, if not otherwise apparent, this paragraph or the next generally should indicate how the letter writer knows the person being written about. Somewhat symmetrically, the closing paragraph should sum up, again identifying the person being written about and the action being recommended. Indeed—like a scientific paper—a letter of evaluation, recommendation, or nomination should have somewhat of an hourglass structure: starting with the big picture, then focusing on details, and finally presenting the big picture again.

APPLICATION ESSAYS, PERSONAL STATEMENTS, AND RELATED WRITINGS

At least in the United States, medical school applicants must submit application essays. Ditto for applicants to other types of health-professional school, to graduate school, and to residency and fellowship programs. And ditto for candidates for some scholarships, awards, and more. Medical editing therefore may include editing various types of application essay (some of which sometimes are known by other terms, such as *personal statements* or *statements of purpose*).

Editing application essays can pose ethical issues, as such writings serve not only to inform readers about the candidate but also to demonstrate the candidate's thinking skills and communication skills. Thus, the substantive editing should not extend to massive rewriting; applicants still should come across as themselves, though now themselves at their best. Accordingly, often it is best to begin by meeting with the applicant, either in person or remotely, to walk through a draft of the essay—answering the applicant's questions, commenting on content and crafting, and requesting clarifications. The applicant then has a basis for revising the draft. Once a revised draft is ready, the editor may help polish it or, if further substantive revision seems advisable, provide more feedback and suggest preparing another draft. In helping to polish application essays, editors should strive to retain the writer's voice, for example by largely maintaining sentence structure and major word choices.

Several problems often appear in drafts of application essays. These problems, and tips for addressing them, include the following:

- *Mismatch with the instructions, prompt, or purpose*: Especially if trying to recycle application essays from other contexts, applicants often provide drafts insufficiently aligned with what is being sought.

A solution is to suggest using the same terms in the essay as in the instructions or prompt, to ensure and demonstrate consistency. For example, if the instructions say to "describe opportunities and challenges," advise the writer to include the words *opportunities* and *challenges* in the opening paragraph, the closing paragraph, and at key points in between. Likewise, if a prompt says to "describe a meaningful experience" or "say how you can contribute to diversity," recommend anchoring the essay with key terms from the prompt.

- *Ambiguity*: Especially because applicants are writing about themselves and their own experiences, they often do not realize what might be unclear to others. For example, they may mention two occurrences and incorrectly assume that readers know the connection. Or they may refer to an event or award just by name, without specifying its nature. (Outside of Texas A&M University, will readers know that Fish Camp is an orientation for incoming students, not a program for anglers or future ichthyologists?) By providing a fresh eye, an editor can help resolve such ambiguities, such as by identifying relationships to make explicit or items to define.
- *Lack of supporting evidence*: Application essays, like much other writing, should largely show rather than tell. Yet drafts of application essays often do too much of the latter and too little of the former. Substantively editing such essays therefore often includes identifying instances where examples or other specifics could supplement or

---

Common Ailments of Medical Application Essays

- Anencephaly: The beginning (head) of the essay is insufficiently developed.
- Osteogenesis imperfecta: The essay lacks a strong unifying structure.
- Dislocations: Some content appears out of place.
  - Type 1: Some content doesn't relate to the paragraph topic.
  - Type 2: Reference is made to material that hasn't been introduced.
  - Type 3: Material is tacked on at the end of the essay.
  - Type 4: Some content doesn't relate to the overall objective.
- Anemia: The essay contains vague statements unsupported by specifics.
- Mermaid syndrome: The end of the essay is insufficiently developed.
- Obesity: The essay is needlessly long, for example because of wordiness.
- Acne: The essay has cosmetic problems (such as errors in grammar, punctuation, or word use).

---

substitute for generalizations. Does an applicant mention having overcome challenges as an immigrant? possessing leadership skills? going above and beyond to help patients? relating well to people from varied backgrounds? being highly devoted to the underserved? If supporting evidence is absent or meager, suggest adding some.

- *Lack of focus*: Drafts of application essays often contain tangents or seem to lack a unifying theme. Therefore, editing them commonly includes helping to increase focus. It may entail helping to identify a unifying theme to make explicit, noting peripheral content to consider deleting, or both; the unifying theme may rightly be as simple as "various experiences have prepared me for this opportunity and shown me that it is a good fit." Occasionally, the current content is so disparate that a major overhaul is advisable. In that instance, talking with the applicant to find a basis for cohesion may especially help.
- *Lack of logical structure*: Substantively editing application essays includes assessing the overall structure. For ease of reading, such essays generally should have a simple, clear structure—for example, chronological or subtopic-by-subtopic. If a draft lacks such a structure or has potentially confusing deviations from it, roles of an editor include suggesting revisions in structure.
- *Poor flow*: Lack of focus and lack of logical structure are two common reasons for poor flow. Other reasons include lack of clear connections between ideas. For instance: Was a second point *in addition* to the first one, *in contrast* to it, or something else? Is it clear where the *first* reason, the *second*, and the *third* each begin? Did something occur *meanwhile* or *next*? Suggesting such transitional words and phrases where warranted, in addition to ensuring that focus and structure are sound, can aid flow and clarity.
- *Ineffective beginning*: Application essays often begin with an overview or anecdote. Either can be effective—or not. If the opening provides an overview of what is to come, editing it entails ensuring that it matches the body of the essay and is concise and clear. Editing an opening presenting an anecdote includes determining whether the anecdote truly seems relevant. (Some applicants incorrectly assume that an anecdote is needed to engage readers.) If the anecdote indeed seems relevant, editing includes ensuring that its relevance is apparent and that the anecdote is clearly and concisely presented.

If an anecdote seems irrelevant or strained, the editor should advise the writer to seek a different anecdote or use a more straightforward beginning.

- *Ineffective ending*: Drafts of application essays often end ineffectively. Sometimes they just stop rather than concluding. Other times, confusingly, the ending mentions a topic not discussed earlier. Normally, the closing paragraph should sum up. If the essay opened with an anecdote, the closing paragraph may well circle back to it in doing so. In any event, the closing paragraph generally should reiterate the main point of the essay. If the closing paragraph mentions a topic not yet discussed, the writer should be advised either to delete the mention or to also discuss the topic earlier.
- *Unsuitable length*: Word count tends to be a bane in writing application essays. Some applicants wonder how they can come up with enough to say. Others wonder how they can condense much of a life into a few hundred words. In advising applicants on drafting such essays, it can be helpful to suggest initially ignoring word count, lest monitoring it result in padding the essay or omitting potentially important information. Once an essay has been drafted, the writer and editor can work together to adjust the length if needed. If an essay is much too short, the writer and editor can identify topics to add or points to develop more. (It is fine, however, for an essay to be slightly below the word limit—for example, 450 words if the limit is 500 words.) If, as is common, a draft is too long, writer and editor can work together to remove less important content, tighten wording, or otherwise condense it.
- *Lack of readability*: Readers of application essays and the like cannot be expected to pore over obscurely written text to extract the meaning. Yet drafts of such essays often are not very readable. In addition to editing for conciseness, items that can increase readability include breaking long, convoluted sentences into shorter, simpler ones; ensuring that paragraphs start with strong topic sentences, so readers stay oriented and the essay is easy to skim; and providing informative opening and closing paragraphs, which aid in previewing and reviewing.
- *Mechanical problems*: Preprofessional students and others writing application essays often have little background in writing. Therefore, their drafts may well have mechanical problems. Spellcheckers and grammar checkers have decreased the number of mechanical

errors in such drafts. However, some mechanical errors—including those of types missed, or even introduced, by such resources—often remain. A common mistake, for example, is for applicants to capitalize the names of diseases. For an application essay to make the best impression, of course it should be polished. Therefore, careful copyediting is advisable.

CVS, RESUMES, AND BIOSKETCHES

An informative, well-crafted *curriculum vitae* (*CV*), resume, or biographical sketch can help health professionals, medical scientists, graduate and professional students, and others obtain employment, grants, honors, and more. It can also aid moderators and hosts in introducing such individuals as speakers. And it can be an important part of an individual's or institution's website. Therefore, professional editing of such items can be highly worthwhile.

A CV and a resume each summarize a person's education and career. However, the length and emphasis tend to differ. A resume generally is the norm in business settings. It typically is limited to one or two pages, and it focuses largely on duties in current and previous employment; these duties usually are presented as bullet points. A CV, which predominates in academia, tends to be considerably longer except for individuals still in training; for mid- and late-career faculty members, it often exceeds 20 pages. CVs include thorough lists of academic achievements, such as journal articles published, grants received, and conference presentations given.

Some people in biomedical fields have both resumes and CVs, for use in different contexts. Some examples of how they can differ: A person's CV might, for example, list dozens of journal articles and several chapters written, but on a resume this publication history might be condensed to "More than 70 articles in journals such as *JAMA*, *Annals of Internal Medicine*, and *Gastroenterology*" and "Chapters in four textbooks of internal medical or gastroenterology." Likewise, a biomedical science instructor's CV might just list taught courses by name, but the corresponding resume might include bullet points listing the duties in each. Also, a person may have different versions of a resume or CV for different purposes, such as applying for research-intensive positions and teaching-intensive ones; the organization and emphasis of the versions may differ accordingly.

Accordingly, one task of an editor can be to help ensure that the provided CV or resume suits the person's objective. Other editing tasks for both CVs and resumes can include checking the following:

- mechanics such as grammar, spelling, and punctuation
- consistency of style and format (examples: whether serial commas are used, how dates are presented, and how headings are formatted)
- parallelism among items in lists
- exactness and conciseness of wording
- clarity (for example, inclusion of an explanatory phrase if the nature of an activity or award may be unclear from its name)

In addition, the editor may advise the author on formatting—for example, inclusion of sufficient white space for readability. An editor also may recommend that the author delete items usually not considered appropriate, at least in the United States, for CVs and resumes in professional biomedical contexts. Such items include the person's marital status, the person's height and weight, and the person's Social Security number (which—believe it or not—commonly appeared in such documents before the emergence of identity theft). Also, unless requested, a photograph of the person normally should not be included. And if a heading has nothing of substance under it, delete the section—lest the person appear like the student who forlornly wrote in her resume, "Honors: None."

Publication lists are a major part of academic CVs. Editing such a CV therefore includes ensuring that publications are listed in an appropriate, consistent format. If a bibliographic format has not been specified, possibilities include that from the National Library of Medicine (Patrias 2007–) or that of a major journal in the person's field. Typically, scientific papers in biomedical fields have multiple authors. In an author list, boldface can be used to make the name of the CV holder stand out. Formatting also can be used to provide other information about the CV holder's role; for example, coauthors who were the person's trainees may have their names italicized, and an asterisk may follow the CV holder's name for articles for which the CV holder was corresponding author. Even if reference management software was used to help prepare the publication list, the editor should check it. Common glitches to watch for include inconsistent capitalization of article titles (with some titles having all major words capitalized and others only the first word and proper nouns capitalized), inconsistent formatting of journal titles (for example, with some titles abbreviated and others written out in full), and problems in spacing.

An editor may also edit *biosketches* (short for *biographical sketches*). In the broad sense, a biosketch is a relatively brief piece of text summarizing a person's experience and qualifications. In ways, it is a narrative version of a resume. Typically, its length ranges from a paragraph to a page. Such biosketches often are posted on individuals' or institutions' websites. They sometimes appear in conference programs or presentation announcements, and sending them to people who will introduce speakers can be helpful. A person may have different versions of their biosketch, with different emphases or lengths, for different purposes. As an editor, you can help ensure that such biosketches are mechanically sound, that they read well, and that they suit their purposes.

In the narrow sense, a biosketch is a document providing, in a required format, specified biographical information on a person seeking a grant or identified in a grant application as part of the proposed project team. For example, the US National Institutes of Health (NIH) requires biosketches, and it provides instructions, templates, and samples for them (National Institutes of Health 2025). By requiring biosketches that provide standardized types of content and that have a standardized format, NIH facilitates the sound, efficient, and equitable review of grant applications. For NIH, biosketches cannot exceed five pages. NIH biosketches include some information, such as that on education and on positions held, that is formatted similarly to that in a CV or resume. They also include narrative portions: a personal statement showing why the person is well suited for the identified role in the proposed project, and descriptions of the person's most significant contributions to science. Of note, whereas a CV usually lists essentially all of a person's publications, an NIH biosketch can cite only a limited number. As an editor, you can help ensure that biosketches such as those for NIH comply with the instructions and are clear, concise, mechanically sound, and persuasive. When editing more than one biosketch for the same grant application, you can also help ensure that the biosketches are consistent with each other and form part of a coherent whole. Because funders revise instructions for biosketches from time to time, take care to consult the most recent ones.

This section on CVs, resumes, and biosketches noted editing such items for conciseness. But how to do so? This question is among those considered in the next chapter, which addresses several aspects of medical manuscript editing not yet explored in this book.

Key Points

- Editing slide presentations and poster presentations tends to include checking for compliance with instructions, streamlining text to promote rapid understanding, assessing suitability of visuals, and checking the mechanics of the writing.
- In editing a conference proceedings or multiauthor text, the editor may be in part a project manager. Keys to success can include early involvement, an organized approach, inclusion of give in the schedule, development of thorough style sheets, and effective communication with authors.
- Editing recommendation and nomination letters commonly includes checking for compliance with requirements, ensuring that sufficient supporting evidence is provided, editing for clarity to intended readers, and condensing text to meet length constraints.
- Editing application essays and related writings requires attention to items such as focus, clarity, flow, and length, as well as mechanics. The editor also should help ensure that the essay begins and ends well.
- Items meriting attention when editing CVs and resumes include consistency of format, parallelism in lists, clarity to intended readers, organization to suit purpose, and inclusion of enough white space.

· 7 ·

Additional Aspects of Medical Manuscript Editing

Excellence as a medical editor often entails skills not only in copyediting or substantive editing per se but also in other areas. This chapter addresses some major such areas. It begins by addressing editing for conciseness, editing for readability, and editing writing by non-native users of English. It also discusses the related skill of proofreading, and it includes points on avoiding overediting and other pitfalls. Finally, it offers guidance on working effectively with authors.

Editing for Conciseness

Drafts of medical writing tend to be wordy. Making them more concise—in other words, making the wording briefer while retaining the meaning—makes them faster and easier to read. Doing so also makes good use of space, a consideration especially when word count or page count is limited, as in abstracts or grant proposals. Five common aspects of editing for conciseness are the following.

(1) *Deleting needless words.* Examples of such deletion include the following:

the field of pediatrics → pediatrics
of an efficient nature → efficient

green in color → green
because of the fact that → because
whether or not → whether
totally destroyed → destroyed

Likewise, in the phrase *entirely unnecessary*, the word *entirely* is unnecessary.

(2) Generally *replacing long words with short synonyms*. Some examples:

attempt → try
currently → now
demonstrate → show
fundamental → basic
numerous → many
subsequently → later
utilize → use

As you may have noticed, these examples regard nontechnical words. In writing for physicians, scientists, and other specialized readers, the medical terminology—which the audience already knows, and which sometimes is more exact—generally should remain. For instance, in writing for general readers, changing *carcinoma* to the shorter, more common term *cancer* may well aid communication. For communication to physicians and scientists, however, this change loses some specificity, as not all cancers are carcinomas.

(3) *Condensing wordy phrases*, as doing so can greatly increase conciseness. Examples:

at the current point in time → now
at some future time → later
in the event that → if
the majority of → most
in most instances → usually
have negative effects on → harm
in a concise manner → concisely

As for the phrase *needless to say*: If something is unnecessary to say, perhaps suggest deleting it.

(4) *Identifying phrases containing nouns derived from verbs, and using the*

verbs instead. Examples of types that arise in medical writing include the following:

produce relief of → relieve
provide an explanation → explain
give a demonstration → demonstrate
have effects on → affect
make contributions → contribute
are dependent on → depend on
are different → differ

(5) In general, *restructuring sentences starting with "There is" or "It is."* For instance, "There is another method that is gaining acceptance" can be condensed to "Another method is gaining acceptance." "There is wide variation in mortality" can be revised to read "Mortality varies widely." And, depending on the context, "It is not necessary to remove this structure" can be recast as either "This structure need not be removed." or "You need not remove this structure."

Decreasing the use of passive voice also can increase conciseness. For example, "The vaccine can be administered by a pharmacist" (eight words) can be condensed to "A pharmacist can administer the vaccine" (six words). However, passive voice need not be totally avoided. When the agent of the action need not be identified (as in the previous sentence and the first part of this one), passive voice is suitably concise.

Finally, *removing double negatives* can increase conciseness or clarity. Some medical authors use wording such as "not unimportant." Did the authors mean "important"? Or did they mean "moderately important"? Querying, and proceeding accordingly, can be worthwhile.

Captions and other text referring to figures or tables often can be shortened by removing mention of the obvious, such as the fact that a given figure is a photograph, and following other editorial tacks. Consider, for example, the statement "Figure 3 is a diagram illustrating a summary of this process." Condensed version: "Figure 3 summarizes this process."

Editing for Conciseness

- Delete unnecessary words.
- Replace long words with short ones.
- Condense wordy phrases.
- Use verbs instead of nouns made from them.
- Restructure sentences starting with "There is."
- Minimize use of passive voice.
- Say what things are, not what they're not.

Beware, though, of altering meaning by removing words that may seem to be redundancies but actually are not. For example, *normal saline* does not just mean an unexceptional solution of salt (sodium chloride); rather, it denotes a particular solution, with a concentration of sodium chloride resembling that in human blood. And do not emulate the editorial trainee who, thinking that of course mice don't wear clothes, removed the *nude* from *nude mice* (a term denoting a particular type of mice used in research). If in doubt whether a seeming redundancy is part of a specialized term, search for the term or query the author.

Appendix 2 ("Words and Expressions to Avoid") in *How to Write and Publish a Scientific Paper* (Gastel and Day 2022, 299–306) presents many more examples of making words or phrases more concise. And "25 Ways to Tighten Your Writing" (Mikel 2015) contains tips that can aid in tightening others' writing as well.

Often, the procedures presented in this part of the chapter can shorten a piece of medical writing at least several percent—without changing content or disrupting flow. The best editing of this type is essentially invisible. Ideally, the text will be briefer and more readable but the author will hardly notice that anything has changed.

Two caveats: *First*, editing for conciseness should aid, not impair, communication—so don't shorten wording at the expense of clarity or accuracy. If the longer wording is the clearer wording, retain it. For example, do not delete transitions or prepositions if they will help readers understand the relationships between ideas, and do not delete *that* if its presence will help avoid misreading a sentence. Don't delete information without the author's permission. And take care to avoid changes that alter meaning. *Second*, especially in editing relatively literary types of medical writing (such as essays, editorials, and book reviews), beware of making changes that increase conciseness but that disrupt rhythm or flow, decrease the richness of the writing, or change the author's voice.

In short, editing for conciseness—like other editing in medicine—requires judgment. Guidelines and principles exist but should not be followed robotically. Thoughtfully done, your editing for conciseness will both save space and save readers' time and effort.

Editing for Readability

Editing thoughtfully for conciseness is part of editing for readability—in other words, refining writing to make it easily understandable on first reading. Editing for readability tends to be especially important in editing medical content for general readers. Such editing also can help ensure that others—such as students, practitioners, and researchers—read, understand, and apply what is written.

Principles of readable writing have long been recognized. For example, *Guidelines for Document Designers*—first published in 1981 (Felker et al. 1981) and then reissued with a new introduction in 2014 (Document Design Project 2014)—presents considerable advice in this regard. In recent decades, readability has gained particular attention through the plain language movement and thus the advent of websites such as plainlanguage.gov (https://www.plainlanguage.gov/) and that of the Center for Plain Language (https://centerforplainlanguage.org/). Principles of *writing* readably can be readily applied to *editing* for readability.

Increasing the readability of medical materials for general readers often includes translating text into simple, common language. Sometimes such editing entails converting specialized medical terms to everyday ones—for example, *hypertension* to *high blood pressure*, *dental caries* to *tooth decay*, *analgesic* to *pain reliever*, or *cerumen* to *earwax*. It also can include replacing highfalutin language—for instance, changing *ambulate* to *walk*, *enumerate* to *count*, or *adjacent to* to *next to*. Many examples in both regards appear in two resources from the US Centers for Disease Control and Prevention: *Everyday Words for Public Health Communication* (https://www.cdc.gov/ccindex/everydaywords/index.html#) and *Plain Language Thesaurus for Health Communications* (https://stacks.cdc.gov/view/cdc/11500). Of course, when knowing technical medical terms may help readers, the terms should be included—but clearly explained. Providing the everyday term before the technical one (example: "bone-building cells, known as *osteoblasts*, and bone-destroying cells, known as *osteoclasts*") often facilitates understanding. Similarly, presenting the concept in simple language and then supplying the technical term can aid readability.

In both technical and nontechnical medical writing, barriers to easy understanding include long sentences, which many in the medical community tend to write. Thus, editing for readability often entails breaking long sentences into two or more sentences apiece. One guideline is to try to limit each sentence to one main idea. Another is to identify sentences that occupy more than two or three lines of a manuscript and consider whether they should be divided. Breaking long paragraphs into more than one paragraph also can aid readability.

Including other elements also can promote readability. Among such elements are the following:

- overviews before details, to help orient readers
- examples (and, when warranted for clarification, "non-examples"—in other words, items that might seem at first to be examples but are not)
- analogies
- narratives, either as brief anecdotes or in longer uses
- visuals such as infographics, diagrams, photographs, maps, and suitably simple graphs

If your role extends to substantive editing, such items can be worth suggesting.

Formatting also can aid readability. Thus, editing for readability may entail adding or improving subheadings, converting run-in lists to bulleted ones, italicizing newly introduced terms, and using (though not overusing) italics or boldface for emphasis. Doing so may also entail, for example, ensuring that a magazine article has multiple *points of entry* (elements that can attract readers). Points of entry may include an engaging title, an informative *deck* (blurb under the title), one or more visuals that draw readers in, and *pull quotes* (short excerpts from the article that are set in larger type). They also may include *sidebars* (short articles accompanying the main article)—for example, a piece explaining some of the science further, a related human-interest piece about a patient or health professional, a glossary, or a list of resources.

Tools to help assess readability include readability checking software such as that included in Microsoft Word. (To turn on this checker, go to "Options" and then "Proofing," and check the box for "Show readability statistics.") Such checkers estimate readability using formulas based largely or solely on word length and sentence length. Commonly, they then express readability in terms of grade level in (US) school. Many providers of medical writing for broad general readerships try not to exceed a sixth- to eighth-grade level; even for educated general readers, keeping text below the tenth- to twelfth-grade level tends to be prudent.

As noted earlier in this book, editors debate—sometimes vehemently—the value of such readability checkers. Opponents note that these checkers fail to consider many factors important to readability, including those as basic as logic; indeed, a passage consisting of brief nonsense sentences consisting of short words would score as very readable. Others of us, while acknowledging the limitations of such scores, find them useful in identifying text that might benefit from simpler language, shorter sentences, or both.

Also, readability scores can aid in persuading authors that editing for readability is warranted. A quantitatively oriented author may be unmoved by an editor's statement that a text would be heavy going even for fellow researchers. Showing the author that a reading score is at the seventh-year postdoctoral level may be more convincing.

Editing Writing by and for Non-Native Users of English

The medical community, and especially the medical research community, is highly international. And English is currently the main international language of science. Thus, editors of medical writing such as journal articles often edit writing by non-native users of English. Some of these authors live and work in predominantly English-speaking countries; others are based elsewhere throughout the world. The authors also vary widely in English proficiency, cultural background, and many other regards. Despite the diversity of this group, a few basic pointers can aid in editing much of the writing by members of this group. (Note: The literature contains a variety of terms for this group. Some authorities favor using *multi-language authors*. However, this chapter will not use this term, as a multi-language author may know multiple languages but not English.)

Dynamics, logistics, and linguistics all can deserve attention when editing writing by non-native users of English. Regarding dynamics: Because such authors are using English as a foreign language, some tend to be especially accepting of English-language editing and especially grateful for it. And the language editing often provides opportunity for substantive editing that further strengthens the work. However, such authors sometimes accept editing too readily, especially if they come from cultures that emphasize showing respect for experts. Thus, if you are unsure whether an edit preserves such an author's intended meaning, asking whether it does so might not suffice; a better option, if feasible, can be to offer two or more versions and ask which (if any) conveys the intended meaning.

Other cultural differences also can be worth considering. For example, some authors come from cultures where attitudes toward time are more casual than those in the United States and United Kingdom.

If such a discrepancy seems likely to exist, expectations for complying with timetables, such as those for submitting revisions to a journal, may deserve discussion. Also, in locales such as some Asian countries, writing tends to be much more indirect than would suit a Western medical journal. For instance, rather than starting with a topic sentence, a paragraph may slowly build up to the main point—or may merely talk around that point, leaving the reader to infer the intended meaning. Accordingly, editors in areas such as the United States or United Kingdom may find the writing to be unfocused, and the authors may feel that some changes by such editors make the writing too blunt and lacking in subtlety. Awareness that cultures sometimes differ regarding directness of communication can yield helpful insights and guidance. For example, rather than being frustrated that a manuscript seems diffuse, editors may realize that a difference in cultural norms may be at play. And they may more quickly realize that reorganizing some passages, adding some topic sentences, and otherwise orienting readers more may help suit the manuscript for its intended venue. Especially if authors may be surprised or dismayed by such changes, explaining the rationale to them can be advisable. A cover letter accompanying an edited manuscript can be a good place to do so.

In some parts of the world, text borrowing that would be considered plagiarism in settings as the United States or the United Kingdom falls within acceptable practice. This discrepancy can lead to problems. A common scenario is as follows:

> You are editing a manuscript by an author who is a non-native user of English. In general, the English in the manuscript is fairly good but not fully idiomatic. One passage, however, is highly polished and not at all in this author's voice. On placing the passage in a search engine, or perhaps using "plagiarism checking" software, you find that the passage is from a published or posted work—perhaps one cited in the manuscript.

You then face the dilemma of how to proceed. Quite possibly, the plagiarism was inadvertent—reflecting such factors as unfamiliarity with relevant norms, difficulty with the language, or carelessness. In any case, a confrontational approach is likely to be inadvisable, especially if the author comes from a culture where maintaining face is important. Rather, noting the relevant norms and working with the author to paraphrase or quote the passage is likely to be most productive and most conducive to promoting a good working relationship.

Regarding logistics: In recent years, technologies have greatly facilitated working with authors overseas. Gone are the days of sending manuscripts between countries by post. And gone are the days of communicating with authors only on paper or through costly international phone calls. With email and other electronic technologies, authors and editors can send manuscripts back and forth almost instantly and quickly exchange comments. Likewise, technologies such as Zoom allow authors and editors to confer face-to-face across the kilometers or miles. Nevertheless, distances can pose challenges. For example, if authors and editors reside in very different time zones, real-time communications can be hard to schedule. However, differences in time zones can be used to advantage; for example, an author may be able to address newly sent queries while the editor is sleeping and then send the answers before the editor's next workday begins.

Regardless of whether an author is remote or local, presenting—or reiterating—key points (for example, regarding schedules) in writing can be especially important if the author has limited English-language ability. Frequently, medical authors overseas read English often for their work but rarely converse in English; they thus tend to understand written English better than spoken English. Also, authors from some cultures hesitate to request clarification even if they do not understand what a speaker says. Presenting key messages in writing helps ensure that the messages are understood and remain available to consult.

Regarding linguistics: Some aspects of English tend to be especially challenging for many non-native speakers of the language. Although areas posing the most difficulty sometimes differ depending on the author's native language, the following tend to be especially common sources of difficulty:

- *Articles*: Some languages do not have the equivalent of the articles *the*, *a*, and *an*. Thus, although proper use of these articles may be intuitive to native speakers of English, knowing when to use them can be difficult for some non-native speakers. Awareness of this difficulty can aid in editing.
- *Prepositions*: Which preposition to use in a given English-language phrase can be seemingly arbitrary. And sometimes analogous phrases in different languages use the equivalent of prepositions with different meanings, thus precluding word-for-word translation. (When I lived in China, I eventually realized that people asking

"May I take a picture for you?" meant "May I take a picture of you?"). Even for native speakers of English, knowing which preposition to use sometimes requires consulting reference works. Awareness that non-native-English-speaking authors can have particular difficulty with prepositions can aid in editing.

- *Verb tenses*: Some languages differ from English in their use of verb tenses. And some languages do not have verb tenses; rather, they indicate timing in other ways. Thus, some non-native users of English have difficulty knowing when and how to use which English-language verb tense. Checking verb tenses can thus be a major part of editing the writing by such authors.
- *Sentence structure*: In English, sentences typically consist of a subject, then a verb, and then an object. Also, in English-language medical and scientific writing, good sentences tend to focus on one main idea apiece and so are relatively short. In some other languages, word order tends to differ from that in English. Also, in some languages, sentences tend to be very long, containing many ideas. In writing in English, some non-native users of the language tend to retain the sentence structure of their native language. Thus, editing their writing can often entail restructuring sentences or dividing sentences into more than one sentence.
- *Capitalization*: Different languages sometimes follow different conventions for capitalization. And some written languages do not have the equivalent of capital and lowercase letters. Therefore, knowing when to capitalize words in English can be challenging to non-native writers of the language, and editors may especially need to revise capitalization in their work.
- *Spacing*: Languages also sometimes differ in conventions regarding spacing, for example relative to punctuation. Therefore, this item too can require particular attention in writing by some non-native users of English.

Increasingly, grammar checkers and related applications of artificial intelligence are helping non-native users of English to avoid some such problems in English-language writing. However, the assistance is not comprehensive, and sometimes the provided changes are incorrect. Thus, although such resources can help authors submit manuscripts that are more polished than otherwise, editing by an editor with full English proficiency remains warranted, just as for manuscripts by native speakers.

Editors who often work with authors with a given native language (such as Chinese or Spanish) tend to become adept at identifying and correcting typical English-language difficulties of these authors. They also may become skillful in guiding authors in avoiding these difficulties. In addition, studying a given foreign language can help an editor in understanding why authors write the way they do, in correcting the resulting errors or infelicities, and in explaining the changes to the authors. Even a brief course in a language or a modest amount of self-study can familiarize an editor enough with the structure of the language to become better at discerning what authors are trying to say and converting the wording to clear, standard English. In addition, studying foreign languages—and perhaps trying to write in them oneself—can provide insight into and compassion regarding the challenges faced by non-native speakers trying to communicate medical content in English.

Knowing the English-language pronunciation patterns of authors with given native languages can aid in discerning what the authors are trying to say. For example, an editing student whose native language was Japanese wrote that she liked the "Glamor Girl" website. After some puzzlement, I realized that she was referring to "Grammar Girl." (By the way, I recommend this website too. It can be accessed at https://www.quickanddirtytips.com/grammar-girl/.)

As well as editing material *by* non-native speakers of English, medical editors often edit English-language materials that are solely or in part *for* readers whose native language is not English or whose culture differs from that of the author or editor. Indeed, given the international nature of the medical community, the audiences for writings such as medical journal articles typically include such readers. Measures to help ensure clarity to such audiences overlap those presented earlier in this chapter for promoting readability. In addition, they include substituting standard, literal language for idioms that may be unfamiliar to readers. They also include advising authors to remove or replace allusions that may baffle readers from other cultures—for example, metaphors based on American football or on cricket, or references to works or cultural figures widely known in only some parts of the world. General sources of guidance in writing, and thus editing, for international audiences include *The Elements of International English Style* by Edmond H. Weiss (Weiss 2005). A journal editorial titled "Writing for the World" (Walshe, Beernart, Chong, et al. 2024) contains advice applicable specifically to editing journal articles to serve readers internationally.

Proofreading: A Related Skill

Non-editors sometimes confuse proofreading and editing. For example, they may ask "Could you proofread my paper?" when in fact they want you to edit the paper. Proofreading, which consists mainly of checking an item for typographical errors, occurs later than editing—either just before an edited item is submitted, once an item is typeset (or the online equivalent) and is nearing release, or both. Editors often are involved in proofreading. For example, an author's editor may proofread a journal article before submission, a manuscript editor at a journal may be involved in checking proofs at the journal, and an author's editor may assist the author in checking proofs that the journal has sent for review.

In addition to addressing typographical errors, proofreading serves as a safety net for identifying serious mechanical errors that went uncorrected during editing. It also can include identifying page-layout problems to correct. Even if text has been carefully edited, typographical errors sometimes sneak in. For example, symbols in the text sometimes mysteriously become something very different. Thus, proofreading includes a sharp eye in this regard. Mechanical errors to be alert for include problems in grammar or punctuation that somehow escaped the editorial eye. Checking proofs of a journal or book also can include watching for deviations from the publication's style—for example, absence of a serial comma from a list if the journal uses serial commas. Accordingly, proofreaders may need to know what style manual is being used, and they sometimes receive the style sheet for the project being proofread. In addition, proofreading includes being alert for inconsistencies in information, such as differences in a number between a table and the text or differences in spelling of a name in different parts of a work.

Regarding the look of proofs: Items to watch for include words in the wrong typeface or type size, problems in spacing, and type that appears misaligned or smudged. Also to be noted are problems of positioning—such as incorrect placement of page numbers or running heads, or poor placement of tables and figures relative to text. In addition, proofreaders should make sure that figures are not upside down, as sometimes occurs, especially if those doing the layout are unfamiliar with medical images. For pieces such as journal articles, make sure the date on the pages is correct. (Sometimes a template has not been updated.) Other items that are considered undesirable, and so should be noted for correction, are *widows* (single lines of text at tops of columns) and *orphans* (single lines of text at bottoms of columns). Ditto for "lakes" or "rivers" (blobs or strips of white space within paragraphs, caused by awkward spacing of words). Proofreaders also should flag figures and tables that appear to be poorly reproduced or whose appearance otherwise seems seriously in need of improvement.

A few more things to look for: Inconsistencies between figures and their captions. Omissions, such as missing references or missing parts of references. Errors in alphabetical or numerical sequence. Incorrect cross-references (such as saying that an item appears in a given section, when in fact it appears elsewhere). Incorrect arithmetic.

With so much to keep track of, how can a proofreader succeed? Checklists can help ensure that proofreading is thorough. Grammar-checking software and related aids also can help. Also, good proofreading generally entails reviewing the text more than once. Looking for different types of problems during different passes through the manuscript can aid in making sure that all problems are noted.

For most of editorial history, proofreading was done on paper manuscripts or printed proofs, using proofreading symbols. For visibility and clarity, changes typically were indicated in colored pencil or colored ink, and they were both marked in the text and designated in the margin. Notes were circled to distinguish them from wording to be inserted. From time to time, occasions still arise to proofread in this way. Lists of standard proofreading marks and examples of their use appear in *The Chicago Manual of Style* (University of Chicago Press Editorial Staff 2024), the *AMA Manual of Style* (AMA Manual of Style Committee 2020), and elsewhere. Other readily accessible lists of proofreading marks include that available at https://www.merriam-webster.com/table/collegiate/proofrea.htm.

Today, materials to proofread usually appear in electronic format, and corrections are to be indicated electronically. For example, article manuscripts and grant proposals to proofread typically arrive in Microsoft Word; corrections can be indicated in Track Changes. Proofs from journals and book publishers generally come as PDF files, with instructions for making corrections using annotation tools in Adobe Acrobat. Even when items to proofread arrive electronically, printing them out to proofread can help, as errors sometimes are difficult to spot onscreen.

Proofreading can entail either only checking a piece for problems such as typographical errors or also ensuring consistency with the previous version. When proofreading a manuscript or proposal before submission, only the former tends to be needed. However, when checking proofs from a journal or book publisher, comparison with the submitted material can be crucial. In other words, depending on the situation, a medical editor may do either *non-comparison proofreading* or *comparison proofreading*.

Non-comparison proofreading entails slow, systematic scrutiny of each word, punctuation mark, and other component (if any) of the item. Reading the item aloud can help, as can having Microsoft Word or other software do so. To avoid distraction by content, some proofreaders not only read the item from beginning to end but also read it backward, either word by word or sentence by sentence.

In comparison proofreading, various approaches can be used to compare the current version (the "live copy") and the previous version (the "dead copy"). Except for very short items, looking back and forth between the two tends to be difficult and ineffective. An approach easier on the eyes and better at detecting discrepancies is to read the dead copy into a recording device and then listen to the recording while looking at the live copy. Another good approach is to have one person read the dead copy aloud while another looks at the live copy; to minimize fatigue, the two can periodically reverse roles. In reading dead copy aloud, not only should every word be pronounced; spellings (for example, of names) should also be read aloud if not obvious, and items such as boldface and italic should be indicated. Also, every punctuation mark should be read aloud, as punctuation can change meaning. (Consider, for example, the following: The phrase "single board-certified pathologist" means "consistently the same board-certified pathologist," whereas "single, board-certified pathologist" [with a comma after *single*] means a pathologist who is unmarried and board-certified.)

If your work as a medical editor includes, or might include, a considerable amount of proofreading, perhaps seek some training specifically in this skill. A variety of guidebooks and freely available online resources on the subject exist, and style manuals such as *The Chicago Manual of Style* provide guidance in this regard. In addition, editorial organizations such as the Editorial Freelancers Association and ACES: The Society for Editing provide materials such as courses or webinars on proofreading. Also, specifically for medical communicators, the American Medical Writers Association offers a workshop on proofreading.

Avoiding Overediting and Other Pitfalls

In medical editing as in much else, more is not always better. In trying to be thorough, medical editors sometimes make excessive changes, follow rules even when doing so runs counter to effective communication, or devote inordinate time to inconsequential details. How do these problems originate? How do they manifest themselves? How can they be avoided? This section addresses such questions, with a few analogies along the way.

Especially to a new editor, thorough editing might seem to require making many changes. However, changes should be made only if the editor can state a reason—such as correctness, clarity, or conciseness. ("I would never have said it that way" is not a valid reason.) Every time a change is made, the risk exists of introducing an error. And changes such as majorly restructuring sentences risk altering the author's voice. An excellent surgeon does the smallest, lowest-risk operation that will solve the patient's problem (and realizes when surgery is not warranted at all). An excellent internist prescribes the most basic, lowest-risk, least expensive medication that will resolve the situation (and knows when not to prescribe a medication at all). Similarly, an excellent editor strives for the simple, small solution and knows when to leave well enough alone.

Some editors and editing companies seem to favor making multiple changes on every page to help show clients that they are receiving their money's worth. However, assurance that writing does not need many changes also is worth obtaining. A medical checkup need not yield a dire diagnosis and extensive treatment plan to be a worthwhile investment. Whether for a patient or a manuscript, a clean bill of health can be a valuable provision.

In *The Subversive Copy Editor* (Saller 2016, 77), Carol Fisher Saller has the following to say to writers:

> You know what it's like to come back to a hotel room in the afternoon and find that housekeeping has been there and everything is all fresh and put to rights? That's how a copy editor would like you to feel when you see the editing. If you can view extra-thorough editing as the mint on the pillow, all the better. What we don't want is for you to feel offended that we saw the need for cleaning.

The extra-thorough editing should not, however, extend to altering the clothes in the closet or replacing them with garments more to the housekeeper's taste. Likewise, those cleaning a home should not take it upon themselves to repaint the walls or remodel the kitchen. In other words, beware of rewriting rather than editing. On spotting a problem, an inexpert editor may tend to rewrite the passage to solve it. Sometimes an expert editor, too, concludes that rewriting is needed. Often, however, an expert editor manages to solve the problem with a deft small change.

In short, the edited version of a piece of writing should still be that piece of writing—but at its best. When we go in for haircuts, most of us want to emerge with our hair looking neater and trimmer and more flattering but still to be clearly recognizable as our hair. And when we have our manuscripts edited, we generally want the muttering in them to be transformed to music but for the music to still be in our voice. For hair, maintaining recognizability may entail keeping the color and texture at least largely the same. For manuscripts, retaining the style may entail largely retaining the main words and general sentence structure while trimming or taming the strays.

As for the pitfall of following rules too rigidly: Much of medical editing does entail following rules—such as those of grammar and punctuation, those of a specific style such as AMA, or those of a particular journal. Yet, these are rules, not laws, and when following them hampers communication, overriding them (or recasting the passage so the issue no longer arises) makes sense. Early in their careers, editors generally are best served by following the rules closely. Later, editors commonly develop a sense of where flexibility exists and what to do when rules are ambiguous or nonexistent. The beginning music student probably should follow the music score closely. The experienced musician has a sense of when and how to syncopate or improvise.

Regarding the third pitfall: The pursuit of perfection sometimes leads editors to spend excessive time trying to resolve details that are inconsequential or beyond their domain. For a medical editor in a staff position, such inefficient use of time may compromise productivity. For a freelancer paid on an hourly basis, it may inflate charges to clients; for a freelancer paid per project, it may yield an inadequate hourly income. The solution depends on the situation.

- *Is a detail of grammar or style of essentially no importance?* If so, just go with one option or another and move on.
- *If an answer hasn't emerged after a reasonable amount of searching, are others likely to have it?* If so, do not feel compelled to be self-sufficient.

Rather, reach out—for example, to your editorial supervisor (if any) or another valued colleague (who may well be flattered to be asked). Especially if the issue might interest others, perhaps pose it in an email discussion list such as that of the Council of Science Editors or an online forum such as the American Medical Writers Association's AMWA Engage.

- *Regardless of your choice, will someone else later have the definitive word?* If so, go with your best guess—and then see how the matter is resolved, so you will know for the future. For example, as an author's editor you may be unable to find clear guidance on how to format an unusual type of reference for the target journal. If so, do not dwell at length on the matter. Rather, format the reference in a way that makes sense and includes all the needed information. Then, if the paper is accepted, those at the journal can decide whether—and if so, how—to reformat the reference.
- *Do you suspect that a fact in a manuscript is incorrect, but you are unable to readily find out for sure?* Remember: A manuscript editor is not expected to be a fact checker. If you suspect that a given fact in a manuscript is incorrect but cannot readily find the answer, query the author, briefly saying why you think there might be an error. The author, who is responsible for the content, can then decide how to proceed.

The conscientiousness and attentiveness to detail that help make for a good medical editor sometimes lead to overediting, excessively rigid compliance with rules, or devotion of disproportionate time to unimportant details. Awareness of these tendencies can help in avoiding them and thus can promote appropriate, efficient editing.

Working Effectively with Authors: The Author-Editor Relationship

Although medical editing is largely a solitary pursuit, it also can be a highly interpersonal one. For instance, you may be an author's editor working with journal articles or grant proposals by medical scientists or health professionals. If so, you may be dealing with hard-won content dear to authors' professional identity and crucial to their professional advancement. Or you may be an editor overseeing work by staff writers or freelance writers. Your authors too may be highly invested in their work and feel they have much at stake. And no matter how proficient authors are as subject experts or professional writers, they may well have insecurities about their text. Accordingly, sensitivity, diplomacy, and tact are in order.

Sensitivity, tact, diplomacy—and respect. A sound and productive author-editor relationship is based on mutual respect. The author is generally a subject expert or professional writer, you're a professional editor, and you and the author should respect each other's expertise. Do not cower or grovel, but do not condescend. Many authors—including medical scientists, health professionals, and writers from journalism backgrounds—are well accustomed to functioning in teams, and showing that you're part of the team can promote effective interaction. Likewise, many authors—perhaps especially clinicians—are well attuned to calling on consultants, and framing yourself as a consultant can be productive.

A good author-editor relationship both eases the editing process and yields a better product. So, what more specifically can you do to work effectively with authors? The following are suggestions to consider.

GENERAL SUGGESTIONS

Regardless of whether you are editing work by a subject expert, a professional writer, or another author, the following measures can promote effective, mutually rewarding interaction.

If applicable, become involved early. If circumstances permit, become a team member or consultant early, while the writing still is being planned. For example, participate in meetings about plans for a grant proposal, or help in planning a scientific paper. Try to remain available for consultation during the writing. Such early participation by editors can facilitate authors' writing and minimize editing later.

Promote a human connection. Especially if you're working remotely from the author, the interaction may tend to be highly impersonal. This situation can suffice, and indeed be most efficient, if the editing will be largely mechanical, such as correcting grammar and punctuation and checking reference formats. However, if the editing will entail deeper engagement with the work, such lack of human connection can be detrimental. Forgetting that a human being is attached to the writing, an editor can too readily be overly heavy-handed in revisions and overly tactless in queries. Introductions—at least in writing and, if feasible, in person, by video call, or by phone—can help editor and author view each other as people and so can help establish the foundation for a good working relationship. Reading about the author also can help. So can posting a photo of the author (for instance, from the author's website) in the corner of your screen when editing the author's work. Also, when wording communications to the author, ask yourself, as author's editor Stephanie Deming recommends (Deming 2010b), "Would I be comfortable in saying this to someone in person?" Such tacks can promote effective interaction.

Put yourself in the author's shoes. Recognize pressures that medical authors might be facing, and that may cause them to be irritable or inaccessible. For example, researchers applying for major grants may have the survival of their laboratories at stake. And clinicians may literally be dealing with life-and-death situations, which clearly take priority over responding to an editor's queries. Also, to promote editorial empathy, remember what it's like to be an author. If you don't like to write, recall why. If you're at least somewhat of a writer yourself, do some writing from time to time. Note how challenging it can be. Observe what it's like to await word about your submission. See how various types of revisions, comments, and queries from editors make you feel. And apply the insights to your interactions with authors.

Coordinate expectations. Authors may not know what the editing will entail. They also may have misconceptions. They may expect the editor to be a meddler who delights in belittling others' writing, not an ally collaborating to help them convey their content effectively and appear their best. Or they may expect the editing to consist just of correcting English, when in fact it may constitute more. Therefore, coordinate expectations. If you have not worked with the author before, explain what you will do and why. Indicate the extent to which your role is advisory. Identify and coordinate timetables; if the editorial process will have successive rounds, indicate them. Provide ample opportunity for authors to ask questions, express concerns, and request attention to specific aspects. Set the stage and the tone for continuing exchange.

Remember that it's the author's piece of writing. As discussed earlier in this chapter, resist the urge to overedit. If something is said acceptably, leave it as is even if you would have said it in another way.

If changes or suggestions may seem questionable, explain them. Sometimes, editing includes making changes or suggestions that may strike authors as odd. For example, the editor may change punctuation to suit a journal's convention that differs from that which the author was taught to use. Or the editor might recommend altering some long-acceptable wording if norms have changed. In such situations, a brief explanation can help keep the author from thinking that the editor is incompetent or that something has gone awry.

Build some give into the schedule. Authors sometimes encounter delays. Ditto for editors. Incorporating some flexibility into the schedule can minimize resulting tensions. In keeping with the maxim "under-promise, but over-deliver," perhaps set schedules such that you will tend to return editing before the target date. If you do experience delays, alert the author as soon as possible. Likewise, encourage authors to alert you of delays, so you can plan accordingly.

If you're angry with an author, cool down. Especially if a strong basis has been established for cordial collaboration, most medical authors are good, or even great, to work with. But sometimes exasperating situations arise: Outlandish last-minute requests. Failure to answer queries or make revisions despite repeated reminders. Seeming obliviousness to potential lapses in ethics. (See next chapter.) Comments that are condescending or downright rude. And more. An editor may well be tempted to lash out with an angry response. But such responses rarely are productive long-term. Take a little time to cool down, and then respond calmly and logically. All will be best served.

Remember to compliment the good. As manuscript editors, we focus on improving the less-than-optimal. Thus, on receiving their edited work, authors may feel that they can do nothing right—even though, in fact, their writing probably has sizeable merits. If work is of overall high quality, say so; or if aspects stand out as especially strong, note them. In communicating with authors, begin and end positively. Not only does such an approach help keep authors from becoming disheartened, but identifying strengths can aid in perpetuating them.

Let the author take the credit. When a journal article, proposal, or popular piece that you helped transform from pitiful to exemplary receives accolades, you may be tempted to say, "But you should have seen it before . . . ." But it is not your role to say so. With luck, the author will laud your contributions. But if not, just stay quiet or say that you're pleased at the success and glad to have been part of the team. Regardless of how much you contributed to shaping the piece, the work is primarily the author's, and you should let the author take the credit.

SUGGESTIONS LARGELY FOR AUTHOR'S EDITORS

A good author-editor relationship can be especially important for author's editors, who mainly help authors improve journal articles, grant proposals, or other materials before submission. Not only can the quality of the product depend in part on the quality of the interaction. Also, unlike a journal's editing of accepted manuscripts, author's editing tends to be optional, and whether an author chooses to obtain it can depend in part on the author's previous interactions with author's editors. Some suggestions for helping author's editors to establish and maintain a productive and cordial relationship with authors therefore follow.

Learn the author's context and concerns. Good author's editing is not a matter of solving a puzzle while using the fewest possible clues. Rather, it should be based on obtaining the best possible information. Therefore, consider taking a little time to obtain some context. Perhaps look at some recent publications by the author. If the author has a website, look at it as well. Maybe have a conversation before editing; in it, perhaps ask how the author became interested in the topic, and perhaps ask the author to summarize the work in nontechnical terms. Of course, if the author hasn't yet specified, find out, for example, what journal will receive the manuscript or what funding source will receive the proposal. Check whether the author would like any parts or aspects to receive particular attention. Also check for other concerns.

Find out any preferences. Some authors have preferences regarding editing received. Whereas queries commonly are presented as comments in Track Changes, an occasional author prefers seeing them in boldface in the text. Some authors want every change to be tracked; others prefer that tracking be limited to substantive changes. And some authors want queries to include full explanations of the request; others just want to know what is being asked for or asked. Collaboration can be aided by giving authors chances to state such preferences, both initially and as feedback on editing received.

If appropriate, serve as an educator. As discussed earlier in this book, authors at different career stages or in different situations sometimes enlist author's editors for different purposes. Busy senior medical researchers sometimes do so largely for efficiency. They may be capable of refining their writing themselves or of learning to do so, but they choose to allocate their time in other ways. And if they have worked extensively with a given author's editor, they may not feel compelled to review every routine change. They may therefore prefer to be relatively unengaged. And indeed, explaining a grammatical change or a query to such an author may come across as condescending. In contrast, for some other types of authors—such as graduate students, medical trainees, postdoctoral fellows, and some visiting international scholars—working with an author's editor serves in part an educational function and so may be approached accordingly. In such a situation, thorough explanations of revisions and queries may be helpful. Likewise, if such authors are unfamiliar with publication procedures or publication ethics, briefing them on relevant aspects or referring them to resources on the subject can fall within the editor's realm.

Return the editing with a helpful cover note. Just as context is warranted at the beginning of an editing project, it is warranted at the end. In returning an edited piece, provide a note that puts it in context. Begin positively; thank the author for the chance to edit the piece, and perhaps note strengths of the writing or say you enjoyed learning about the topic. (Complimenting the author on the research itself, however, may come across as insincere unless you are an expert on the topic.) Then provide an overview of the editing done—for instance, summarizing types of revisions made, providing general queries or overall suggestions if relevant, and perhaps explaining aspects of the editing that the author might wonder about. This part of the note can vary considerably in length. Especially if the editing is routine and you have worked with the author before, a paragraph or just a sentence may suffice. In other instances, such as when "educationally editing" a scientific paper by an inexperienced author, it might run a couple of pages and include a paragraph on each major section of the paper. Finally, the note should end positively, for instance by thanking the author again, noting availability to answer questions, and, if applicable, saying you hope to work with the author again.

Consider providing both a tracked manuscript and a copy with all changes accepted. If a manuscript has many copyeditorial revisions, the author may initially find the tracked version overwhelming. If such may be the case, consider also providing a copy without tracking and suggesting that the author look at it first to get an overall sense of the edited version.

Consider following up. Perhaps also follow up on the editing. For example, if you see that a paper you edited has been published or a grant for which you edited the proposal has been funded, congratulate the author. Doing so can cultivate an ongoing good working relationship and help generate future work.

SUGGESTIONS LARGELY FOR COMMISSIONING EDITORS

Perhaps you assign and edit medical writing for a magazine, newsletter, blog, or website. Or perhaps you oversee writing and revision of news releases for an institution. In such situations, the following guidance can help.

Respond quickly and constructively to pitches. In some settings, you may receive article proposals (commonly referred to as *pitches* or *query letters*) from freelance writers. Or, if you have staff members, you may receive article ideas from them. In either case, try to respond promptly, so the person knows whether to proceed. If a freelancer impresses you but you decide not to accept the current story idea, consider encouraging them to submit future pitches—or perhaps offer the freelancer a story you have been wanting to find someone to write. Similarly, if a staff member's idea does not suit, express appreciation nevertheless, and perhaps guide the

---

Sample Message Accompanying Edited Manuscript Returned by Author's Editor

Dear Dr. _____:

Thank you for the opportunity to edit your paper, "_______." I enjoyed learning about this research and appreciated how well the paper was organized. In keeping with our discussion, I have edited the manuscript to comply with the instructions from the *Journal of Medical* ______.

As discussed when we spoke, I have edited the manuscript in Track Changes. Suggested revisions are provided within the text, and comments and queries appear in bubbles next to it. Please review my edits to ensure that I have retained your intended meaning. Of course, you are free to accept, reject, or modify my edits.

You might notice that I have replaced the term ______ with the term _______. I have done so in keeping with new guidance released last month by the *AMA Manual of Style*.

In reviewing the paper, I noticed that it contained more figures and tables than the maximum stated in the journal's instructions to authors. Perhaps you could submit some of them as supplementary materials. Also, the manuscript did not seem to include a paragraph on limitations, as is typical in the journal. If you add such a paragraph, I would be glad to edit it.

Again, thank you for the chance to edit your paper. If you have questions, please feel free to ask. I wish you all the best with publication of this paper and hope you will call on me again.

Edie Editor

---

staffer in reshaping the idea or understanding what kinds of ideas are being sought. If an idea is accepted, guide the freelancer or staffer in pursuing (and, if needed, adapting) the idea, to maximize likelihood that the piece meets your needs without rewriting or extensive editing.

If initiating work, try to match authors (and others) with the assignments that best suit them. As an editor, you may assign staff or freelance writers to stories you want written. For best results, try to match people with types of stories for which they are best qualified and that they enjoy the most. For example, some medical writers have extensive basic-science background and thrive mainly on writing about laboratory research. Others struggle with covering such research but are in their element writing human-interest medical stories or pet-related veterinary stories. Matching writers and stories accordingly—or having writers collaborate on stories that draw on their respective strengths—can yield the best product and most satisfied writers. Similar principles are worth following when enlisting illustrators, photographers, and others—including manuscript editors if you will not be copyediting stories yourself.

Make expectations explicit, and, if relevant, provide guidance in achieving them. To minimize miscommunication, put expectations—regarding length, deadlines, and other items—in writing. At some publications, contracts are provided in this regard. In some other settings, an email message suffices. If warranted, also provide guidance in preparing the story you envision. For example, if you know of people to consider interviewing, note them and provide their contact information. Or if a previous story could serve as a model for the current one, provide it. Retain some flexibility, as stories sometimes develop in unexpected directions—but inform the writer to alert you if a story seems to be evolving in a way other than initially envisioned.

Within reason, adapt to authors' working styles. Some authors are happiest and produce their best work if the editor checks in periodically between making the assignment and receiving the finished story. Others prefer to proceed on their own—and indeed might be annoyed by such check-ins—but likewise provide suitable work on time. Then there's the occasional author who is exceptionally able but chronically late; editors learn to build extra give into schedules when working with them. When working repeatedly with the same authors, knowing and adapting to their working styles can help yield the best product and smoothest interaction.

Promptly acknowledge submissions. "Did the story arrive? And is it OK?" even experienced authors may worry. So, promptly acknowledge receipt. If feasible, also give the material a quick read and, barring indications otherwise, an overall positive word. Perhaps also take the opportunity to state, or reiterate, what the next steps will be.

Consider asking questions rather than making criticisms or corrections. If you perceive aspects of a piece as unsuitable, the easiest tack can be to criticize them or do some rewriting. Sometimes, however, a better approach is to ask questions that help the author perceive the difficulty and recognize how to resolve it. For example, you might ask "Does this list seem to be in the most logical order?," "Will readers understand these terms?," "Is it clear enough how this point supports this conclusion?," or "Might it be helpful to add ____?" The author can then make the revisions—maintaining the voice of the writing, retaining a sense of ownership of the piece, and perhaps learning along the way.

Especially if the writer will continue submitting work to you, try to be a teacher or coach. In keeping with the previous point, try to help authors continue developing their skills. For example, explain revisions for which the reasons might not be obvious. And perhaps share or suggest resources that might be helpful. Such measures can cultivate a collaborative relationship, and in the long run they can save time.

Be specific in your suggestions. Vague requests such as "Make this clearer" or "Make this more interesting" may baffle and frustrate an author, who may think an item already is clear or interesting (or who may suspect that it is confusing or boring but be at a loss about what to do about it). Try to identify the problem more exactly and suggest how to resolve it. Then, for example, you might say "To make this paragraph clearer, please state the relationship between ___ and ___." or "To make this part of the article more interesting, please try to add a quote from the researcher, the story of a patient who benefited, or ideally both."

If doing so might help, provide guidance in carrying out suggestions. If authors may be unsure how to pursue suggestions such as those for further developing their stories, provide guidance. Examples include noting written sources of information, providing names and contact information of additional experts to consider interviewing, and identifying institutions and organizations that may be able to connect writers with patients or family members.

When working with freelancers, strive to ensure prompt payment. More broadly, advocate for the compensation and recognition of those writing for you. Work with your business office or other relevant unit to ensure that freelancers are paid without delay. Likewise, advocate for raises and promotions of deserving writers on staff. Also advocate for professional-development activities, such as conference attendance, for the staff. When appropriate, nominate writers or their work for awards, such as those from the Association of Health Care Journalists, the National Association of Science Writers, and the Council for the Advancement of Science Writing. Regardless of how busy you might be, remember to compliment writers on excellent work and to let them know that they are appreciated. As well as being the right thing to do, such measures cultivate productive working relationships with—and loyalty from—writers.

FOR MORE ON THE AUTHOR-EDITOR RELATIONSHIP

A set of insightful, engaging articles on fostering an effective author-editor relationship, especially as an author's editor, appeared in *Science Editor* (the periodical of the Council of Science Editors) from 2009 to 2011 as a series titled "Between Author and Editor." Especially recommended articles from this series include "Starting Off on the Right Foot" (Deming 2009a), "Some Prescriptions for Better Editor-Author Communication" (Deming 2010a), and "Queries: Conversing with the Author in Writing" (Deming 2010b)—all by Stephanie Deming, longtime substantive editor at the University of Texas MD Anderson Cancer Center, who oversaw the series. Some articles in this series can be accessed from *Science Editor* (https://www.csescienceeditor.org/). Later articles on the topic include the Council of Science Editors annual meeting report "Collaborative Copyediting: Helping the Author Help You" (DiAngelis 2023).

Key Points

- Editing for conciseness facilitates reading and helps make good use of space. Aspects of such editing include deleting needless words, replacing long words with short ones, condensing wordy phrases, and using verbs instead of nouns derived from them.
- Editing for readability commonly includes, in addition to increasing conciseness, such items as replacing specialized medical terms with everyday language where warranted, breaking up long sentences and paragraphs, adding overviews, suggesting addition of easy-to-understand visuals, and providing formatting such as subheadings and bullets.
- Editing medical writing by non-native users of English entails

considering both culture and language. Existence of different cultural norms (for example, for organizing communications) can be worth keeping in mind. So can aspects of English with which non-native users often have difficulty (for example, articles such as *the* and *a*, prepositions, verb tenses, sentence structure, and capitalization).

- Proofreading can include checking for typographical errors, noting mechanical errors missed during editing, and identifying problems in layout.
- Among pitfalls to avoid in editing are making excessive changes, following rules rigidly even if communication suffers, and devoting inordinate time to inconsequential details.
- Effective author-editor relationships are important, especially for author's editors and for editors who commission writing. General suggestions in this regard include promoting a human connection, considering the author's perspective and proceeding accordingly, and coordinating expectations.

· EXERCISE ·

Editing for Conciseness

Condense the wordy part of each of the following sentences. Do not make other changes. Take care not to change meaning.

1. The majority of nurses report this problem.
2. They completed the task in an efficient manner.
3. Editing has the potential to improve text.
4. The procedure produced an increase in the rate.
5. Despite the fact that he took the course, he edits poorly.
6. Next we counted the number of cells.
7. Patients of many different nationalities attend the clinic.
8. The lesion was green in color.
9. She discussed advances in the field of neurology.
10. They should exercise on a daily basis.

· 8 ·

Ethics

YOUR OWN AND OTHERS'

Because medical research and medical information affect health and well-being, ethical practices in medical writing, editing, and publishing are literally vital. Thus, complying with professional ethics is especially important for medical editors. In addition, medical editors help ensure that authors follow ethical practices. This chapter therefore both summarizes ethical obligations of medical editors and provides a foundation for serving as a resource for authors regarding publication ethics.

Underlying Principles

Various principles underlie ethical behavior in medical editing, medicine, and medical science. These principles, in turn, derive from a mix of approaches or perspectives. Some come from rules-based (deontological) approaches. Others are outcome-based (teleological). Others come from other standpoints, such as those prioritizing quality of human relationships. For medical editors, and for others involved in communicating medicine, key principles tend to include the following:

- *Veracity*: Clearly, medical communication must be truthful. Medical editors must maintain the accuracy of what they edit, obtain clarification if they suspect inaccuracy, and seek correction if content indeed seems inaccurate.

- *Trustworthiness*: Medical editors must be responsible. They need to do what they say they will do. They also must strive for excellence in their work.
- *Transparency*: Medical editors need to promote full and accurate disclosure of items such as funding sources of research being reported and authors' roles in the research and writing. They need to avoid or report conflicts of interest, and they should help ensure that authors disclose such conflicts. They also should be transparent about their own limitations.
- *Confidentiality*: Medical editors often deal with confidential information, such as unpublished research results. They must take care to maintain its confidentiality.
- *Beneficence*: An overriding principle is to do good. Editorial changes should be made only if they will improve the product. They should not just reflect personal preference. More broadly, editors' actions should promote the quality of writing and the well-being of authors.
- *Nonmaleficence*: As is often said in medicine, "First, do no harm." Editorial changes should not introduce errors or otherwise impair the product. More broadly, editors' actions, including those to address ethical issues, should not lead to undue harm.
- *Autonomy*: Editors should respect the free will of authors. Insofar as conditions permit, they should let the authors make the final decisions.
- *Respect*: As well as supporting authors' autonomy, editors should show respect for authors in other regards. They should respect authors' subject-matter expertise, refrain from demeaning authors' writing, and strive to understand and adapt to authors' priorities and constraints.
- *Justice*: Editors should be fair in their interactions. They should not favor some authors over others. Likewise, they should not arbitrarily favor certain colleagues or subordinates in their work.
- *Universalizability*: Editors should strive to be consistent in their dealings. They should try to limit exceptions other than in situations where other principles are of overriding importance.
- *Rationality*: Editors should be able to state reasons for their decisions. Justifications such as "it just felt right" or "it just didn't feel right" should not suffice.

Ethical dilemmas can arise if, for example, different principles favor different courses of action. The last section of this chapter will discuss approaching such dilemmas. But first, largely based on these principles, this chapter will discuss proceeding ethically as a medical editor.

Ethical Obligations of Medical Editors

Medical editors have a variety of ethical obligations, including some relating to their interactions with authors and some regarding the integrity of their work. Based in part on an excellent list (Young 1997) presented at a meeting of the Council of Biology Editors (the forerunner of the Council of Science Editors), the current section focuses primarily on ethical obligations of medical manuscript editors. Much of the content, however, also applies to professional medical editors in other roles. Lists of principles to follow include the Board of Editors in the Life Sciences Code of Ethics (Board of Editors in the Life Sciences 2024) and more generally the American Medical Writers Association Code of Ethics (American Medical Writers Association, n.d.), on which the former is in part based.

A basic obligation is to *maintain confidentiality*. A manuscript for a medical journal is confidential. Prematurely sharing its content can have serious repercussions, such as giving undue advantage to the author's competitors, releasing health-related conclusions not yet vetted for validity, and posing problems regarding commercialization or investment. Likewise, a grant proposal is confidential, and sharing content from it may lead to others' stealing ideas. Thus, unless the author has given permission, editors of such documents should not share them or discuss the content with others. Likewise, editors should not gossip about the quality of the writing; the prize researcher or the dean might have provided a manuscript riddled with grammatical errors, but that fact is not for others to know. And if medical editors are professionally privy to confidential information about patients, research participants, trainees, or others, of course they should not share it.

If a medical editor works in an office serving multiple authors, another principle is to *avoid favoritism*. You may be tempted to lavish attention on writing by an author who is polite and appreciative and brings you candy or flowers. And you may wish to devote minimal effort to that of the author who is gruff, acts entitled, and maybe could benefit from more frequent showers. But every author's work deserves equally thorough editing. If you are a freelance editor and your resources allow, you may refuse work from authors you dislike. If, however, you accept their work, it should receive the same high quality of editing as the rest. And when—for whatever purpose—you turn down work, good professional practice is to help the author find a suitably qualified editor; options include recommending specific editors and referring the authors to freelance directories such as those of the Board of Editors in the Life Sciences and the American Medical Writers Association.

Speaking of bringing you candy or flowers: Small tokens of appreciation such as these can be appropriate to accept. However, large or highly personal gifts (one medical editor tells of receiving a gift certificate to a lingerie store!) can be awkward at best, especially as they might at least seem to be currying editorial or other favoritism. Such gifts are best graciously declined, for example with a statement that the gratitude is much appreciated but the gift must be refused, in keeping with norms in the field. Some institutions where medical editors work have policies regarding the size and nature of gifts that employees may accept; of course, these policies should be followed. Sometimes an appropriate tack is to share a gift, such as a fruit basket, with colleagues or to donate a (less perishable) gift to charity.

Although authors' conflicts of interest receive more attention, editors likewise need to *avoid conflicts of interest or be transparent about them*. Contrary to a common misconception, having a conflict of interest does not mean being biased; it simply means being in a situation that can predispose to bias. Such situations are best avoided, or at least disclosed. If editors suspect that they risk introducing bias when editing given manuscripts—for example, because they feel strongly about the topic or have invested in a company whose stock prices might be affected by a publication—they should decline the editing or they should reveal the conflict, so the author or the editor's supervisor can decide whether to proceed. Likewise, a freelance editor should beware of accepting work from a competitor of a client currently being served.

In keeping with avoiding conflicts of interest, editors should *avoid and counter overstatement*. Perhaps unconsciously, authors of journal articles sometimes overstate implications of their findings. Also, public information staff members writing news releases sometimes overstate the benefits of a medical advance, either because they misinterpret the science or because they think doing so will help their institution or company. Indeed, editors themselves may be tempted to overplay content for this purpose. However, such overstatement is dishonest, and it can backfire. Ditto for overstating the editor's qualifications and for accepting work with aspects beyond the editor's expertise without stating the limitations of what can be provided. (Example of such a statement: "As a substantive editor with an MD, I can provide some editorial assistance with this dental manuscript, but my feedback on content might not be as thorough as that on a medical manuscript. Would you like me to proceed anyway, or would you like me to help you find an editor with a background in dental editing?")

Two other ethical obligations entail being sure to query when uncertainty arises about accuracy of content. To avoid introducing errors, editors need to *query the author when proposing revisions that might change meaning*—for example, a major rewording of a passage or a change intended to remedy what seemed to be an incorrect fact. Also *query the author about conclusions that seem unsupported by the evidence presented.* Although the latter can require particular tact, it can be important to the integrity of the piece.

Another ethical obligation is to *stay up-to-date in the field.* Over the years, norms in general and in medical editing evolve, editorially relevant technologies advance, new information sources for editors emerge, and more. Therefore, to maintain excellence in their work, medical editors need to stay current. Fortunately, professional societies, continuing-education opportunities, publications, and other resources can aid in this regard.

Finally, an obligation of medical editors is to *educate authors about ethical publication practices.* Some editors, such as some at medical institutions, provide formal training on this subject. Regardless of the setting, medical editors should be versed in basics of medical publication ethics and ready to provide guidance in this regard. Such basics are the topic of the next section.

Editors as Resources Regarding Medical Authors' Ethics

Medical manuscript editors are not the ethics police. They are not expected to scrutinize every document in search of indications that ethical violations have occurred. Rather, they should approach their work with the assumption that, barring evidence otherwise, authors have acted ethically. Sometimes, however, an author is unaware how to proceed. And sometimes clues exist that an author might have acted, perhaps inadvertently, in a way inconsistent with publication ethics. Accordingly, the editor should be able to answer questions about publication ethics, refer authors to resources on the topic, and, if problems may exist, take next steps.

Integrity in research—and thus in research publication—includes, of course, avoiding *fabrication* (making up findings), *falsification* (changing findings or omitting relevant ones), and *plagiarism* (passing off others' words or ideas as one's own) (Office of Research Integrity, n.d.). Of these problems, the one that medical editors encounter most often is plagiarism. In a document, plagiarized work commonly appears as a passage that differs in style from the rest of the text or that appears to lack a citation. Often, the plagiarism seems to be inadvertent, reflecting carelessness in writing, unfamiliarity with proper citation practices, or cultural differences in what is permissible to take from others' work. Tactfully exploring the situation with the author—and, if plagiarism has occurred, helping the author to correct the problem and understand how to avoid future such problems—can often resolve the situation.

A manuscript editor is less likely to detect and deal with fabrication or falsification. Clues, though, that such problems might exist include data that appear too nearly perfect, findings that seem to have been generated unrealistically fast (for example, almost instantly after a peer reviewer requests an additional experiment), omission of relevant data that presumably would have been collected, and inclusion of images that seem to be the same as in a previous paper. An unconfrontational discussion with the author may resolve the situation, for example by showing that the suspicions are unfounded or eliciting inclusion of missing information. Otherwise, sound practice tends to entail reporting the concerns to someone appropriately situated to decide whether to explore the situation further—for example, your supervisor (if any), the author's supervisor, or the research integrity office at the author's institution.

Much medical investigation, of course, includes humans or animals as research subjects, rather than being restricted to the test tube or computer or the like. As mandated by law, research on humans must be approved as ethical by an *institutional review board* (commonly known as an IRB) before being conducted; that on animals must be approved by an *institutional animal care and use committee* (generally referred to as an IACUC). And, to be considered for acceptance, journal submissions must document these approvals. Editors' roles can include ensuring that manuscripts note the approvals. Also, editors sometimes help refine required documents such as the applications for approval and the forms for obtaining human participants' informed consent to take part in the research. Editors also can help educate authors about such matters—

including the need for approval even if, for example, people being studied are asked only to complete a questionnaire.

Unless indicated otherwise, medical writing must be *original*. One aspect, of course, is avoiding plagiarism. Another is avoiding *duplicate publication*, such as publication of the same paper in more than one journal. If a paper is to be republished—for example, in translation—it must be clearly identified as a republication. Questions relating to originality of wording sometimes arise regarding papers that report new findings but draw on previously reported methods. Examples include successive papers from longitudinal studies that follow the same people for many years or from large, multifaceted studies that generate different papers on different aspects. If methods are the same, either in a study over time or in different studies of the same type, few ways of describing them may exist. In such situations, what has come to be known as *text recycling* can be acceptable. Norms regarding text recycling are evolving. Sources of current information include the Text Recycling Research Project (https://textrecycling.org/). A conference-session summary in *Science Editor* (Isaacson 2023) briefs editors on text recycling.

If a study is indeed long or multifaceted, it may validly generate multiple papers. Sometimes, though, authors hoping to advance their careers by publishing many papers try to derive more than one paper from even a small study—for example, by presenting some of the findings in one paper and the rest in another, although the findings would most logically and helpfully appear in a single paper. Such thin slicing of results—sometimes termed *salami science* (or perhaps better *cucumber science*, so as not to exclude vegetarians)—tends not to serve readers well. It also may backfire for the authors, as a paper presenting all the findings may be accepted by a more prestigious journal and advance the authors' careers more than two papers in a less prestigious journal. Editors who notice possible attempts at salami science may aid authors and readers by suggesting that the publication strategy be reconsidered.

Medical research typically entails the work of multiple people, with contributions of varied types and sizes. Therefore, whom to list as a paper's authors can lead to uncertainty and contention. Accordingly, in medical publication ethics, *authorship* has been a major area of discussion. The upshot of the discussion is that the names on the author list should be those of the individuals with substantial intellectual input into the research. The list should not include people with little or no such input (*guest authors*). Nor should there be *ghost authors*: people who merit authorship but whose names are omitted. Also, it should be remembered that authorship signifies not only credit for the work but also responsibility for it.

As discussed in earlier chapters: Many medical journals use the authorship criteria specified by the International Committee of Medical Journal Editors, commonly known as the ICMJE (International Committee of Medical Journal Editors, n.d.), or similar criteria. In addition, some require that submissions specify *contributors*—in other words, say who contributed to which aspect(s) of the work. If an editor either sees that someone in the author list has no contributions listed or notices a key contribution for which no one is identified, the editor should alert the main author to the discrepancy, so that appropriate corrections can be made.

For an author's editor, roles relating to authorship and contributorship can include educating early-career researchers about relevant norms and answering questions in this regard. Longstanding (and periodically updated) resources to call on include the portion of the ICMJE website that addresses this topic (https://www.icmje.org/recommendations/browse/roles-and-responsibilities/defining-the-role-of-authors-and-contributors.html), the authorship part of the ethics chapter in the *AMA Manual of Style* (AMA Manual of Style Committee 2020, 172–91), and the authorship section of the Council of Science Editors *Recommendations for Promoting Integrity in Scientific Journal Publications* (Council of Science Editors Editorial Policy Committee, n.d.). In addition, *Authors Without Borders: Guidelines for Discussing Authorship with Collaborators* (Bird, Hosseini, and Plemmons 2023) can facilitate authorship discussions not only among researchers but also between editors and researchers.

In recent years, the following question has arisen: If artificial intelligence (AI) has been used in writing a paper or doing the research on which it is based, should the AI tool be listed as an author? The consensus among authorities is that an AI tool should not be listed as an author, in part because it cannot take ethical responsibility for the work. The use of AI should, however, be identified and described. Typically, this information should appear in the methods section of the paper. In the case of minor contributions, it may appear in the acknowledgments.

When author's editors markedly improve papers, grateful authors sometimes offer to add them to the author list. However, unless (as is very rare) the editor's contributions meet the criteria for authorship, the offer should—gratefully and graciously—be declined. Nonetheless, such editing, especially if substantive, should be noted in the contributions list, acknowledgments, or both. Acknowledging editorial assistance is part of *transparency*. Indeed, to help ensure such transparency, some editors or editorial offices routinely add a brief acknowledgment—such as "We thank Eddie Editor for editorial assistance" or "Ellie Editor provided scientific editing services"—to manuscripts they edit. (Normally, editing at the journal is not acknowledged, as publication there already discloses that the paper has received editorial attention from its staff.)

Other aspects of transparency include authors' disclosing *conflicts of interest*, such as financial ties to companies whose products they study, and identifying *funding sources* of research being reported. Editors can help ensure that journal submissions include this information and that it is accurate and complete. Some authors do not realize that a conflict of interest is defined by the potential of a situation to affect judgment, not whether they think it affected their judgment. And sometimes they believe, incorrectly, that disclosing conflicts of interest will preclude publication. Educational roles of medical editors can include countering such misperceptions.

A medical editor also should help ensure compliance with *confidentiality*, *anonymity*, and related ethical norms. Doing so includes, for example, making sure that case reports are submitted for publication only with permission of the patient or an appropriate surrogate; that photographs of patients and research participants are published only with their permission (or that the photos contain nothing from which the individuals could be identified); and that articles for the public include medical information about specific people only with their permission. In veterinary contexts, needed permissions should be obtained from the animal's owner or other person responsible.

In peer review, maintaining confidentiality and disclosing conflicts of interest also are tenets. Submissions to journals are privileged communications, and peer reviewers are not to share or discuss them with others without the journal's permission. Also, those invited to peer-review papers must disclose any possible conflicts of interest regarding the submission, after which the journal decides whether to proceed with the review. At a journal, a medical editor may be involved in communicating such norms to authors and helping to see that the norms are followed. In institutional settings, author's editors may take part in educating authors about such norms.

Medical publication ethics is a large and complex topic; this section has just touched on some main aspects medical editors may encounter. Fortunately, sources of extensive information and guidance exist regarding ethics of authors, editors, peer reviewers, and publishers. Prominent such sources include the Council of Science Editors *Recommendations for Promoting Integrity in Scientific Journal Publications* (Council of Science Editors Editorial Policy Committee, n.d.), known in its initial versions as the "CSE White Paper on Publication Ethics"; the ICMJE "Recommendations for the Conduct, Reporting, Editing, and Publication of Scholarly Work in Medical Journals" (International Committee of Medical Journal Editors 2024); the chapter "Ethical and Legal Considerations" in the *AMA Manual of Style* (AMA Manual of Style Committee 2020, 171–409); and the COPE (Committee on Publication Ethics) website (https://publicationethics.org/). The COPE website contains multiple types of materials, including guidelines, cases, and educational items, as well as flowcharts indicating how best to proceed in a variety of situations. For brief, readable overviews of research ethics, including publication ethics and other aspects, excellent resources include *On Being a Scientist: A Guide to Responsible Conduct in Research* (Committee on Science, Engineering, and Public Policy 2009) and *Doing Global Science: A Guide to Responsible Conduct in the Global Research Enterprise* (InterAcademy Partnership 2016); both books are openly available online.

Additional resources include those detailing and discussing misconduct in medical and scientific research and publication. One such resource is the well-developed blog Retraction Watch (https://retractionwatch.com/), which reports on retractions of scientific papers and on related topics. (Note, however, that not all retractions of journal articles occur because of misconduct. Sometimes fine researchers discover serious problems in their studies after publication and so, in keeping with scientific integrity, withdraw the papers reporting them.) Publishers also can be valuable sources of such information. For example, a fellow editor has noted a helpful series from the publisher Elsevier on detecting papers from "paper mills," which would-be authors pay to fabricate papers in their names (https://www.elsevier.com/connect/paper-mills-see-the-wood-for-the-trees-part-1, https://www.elsevier.com/connect/paper-mills-see-the-wood-for-the-trees-part-2, and https://www.elsevier.com/connect/paper-mills-see-the-wood-for-the-trees-part-3). Medical editors working in contexts where fraudulent papers or other misconduct seems likely to be encountered may find it especially useful to keep up with such resources.

Approaching Ethical Issues

So, an ethical concern has arisen. Perhaps you are wondering how to proceed most ethically in some aspect of your own work. Or perhaps you suspect that an author is proceeding unethically or is on the verge of doing so. How best to approach such quandaries? Three basics to keep in mind are to gather and reflect on information, assume good intent, and involve others if warranted.

Your intuition can be a good place to start in determining whether an ethical quandary exists. Such feelings should definitely not be neglected. But of course, involve your intellect as well. In keeping with earlier in this chapter, consider ethical principles, potential outcomes, and relationships with those involved. If warranted, review parts of this chapter, consult resources such as those noted at the end of the previous section, and look at additional materials offered by organizations in relevant fields. Also realize that you have a professional community, some members of which might well already have confronted or considered the situation you are facing. While taking care not to violate confidentiality if the issue regards behavior of someone other than yourself, make use of that community. Consider consulting a supervisor, mentor, or wise colleague. Also consider bringing questions to the email discussion list or online forum of a professional organization such as the Council of Science Editors or the American Medical Writers Association; as well as providing perspectives for you to consider, the discussion may aid others. Then, if the situation permits, take some time to reflect on what you have found.

If you think an action by an author may be questionable, do not assume ill intent, and do not approach the author confrontationally. Rather, state your observation (for example, "This wording seemed very similar to . . ." or "No conflicts of interest are listed, but I thought I recalled . . ."), and request more information. Your observation might be incorrect, or a valid reason might exist for what you observed. Alternatively, the author might lack suf-

Some Resources on Publication Ethics—and on Lack Thereof

- *Recommendations for Promoting Integrity in Scientific Journal Publications* (from the Council of Science Editors)
- "Recommendations for the Conduct, Reporting, Editing, and Publication of Scholarly Work in Medical Journals" (from the International Committee of Medical Journal Editors)
- "Ethical and Legal Considerations" (in the *AMA Manual of Style*)
- COPE (Committee on Publication Ethics)
- Retraction Watch

ficient knowledge about the norms, in which case you can provide some briefing and work with the author to avert an undesirable situation. If the author was indeed trying to violate ethical norms, such an approach can allow the author to correct the actions while still saving face. Only if evidence of a possible problem remains would the situation be brought to the attention of those at a higher level. A similar approach is warranted in the (rare, one hopes) instance that one suspects that a fellow medical editor is not following best ethical practices.

If suspicion remains of unethical conduct by an author or other, inform someone who has responsibility for such matters. As noted earlier, manuscript editors are not the ethics police, and it is not their role to investigate possible wrongdoing. Rather, as concerned citizens of the medical communication community, they should bring suspicions to those whose duty includes deciding how to proceed when such concerns arise. Depending on your setting, such a party may, for example, be your editorial supervisor, an editor-in-chief, the supervisor of the individual concerned, or an ethics office at the individual's institution.

Fortunately, most medical editors rarely encounter serious ethical infractions. And commonly, ethical issues that do arise tend to reflect readily resolvable misunderstandings of norms. With basic knowledge of principles, norms, resources, and procedures, medical editors can approach ethical issues with minimal stress and maximal success.

Exemplary medical editors both behave ethically and serve as resources regarding the ethics of others involved in medical writing and publication. Beyond avoiding misconduct and preventing or countering that by others, they embody integrity by fulfilling their obligation to promote excellence in medical writing, editing, and publication. It is hoped that this chapter and others in this book aid in these pursuits.

Key Points

- Key ethical principles for medical editors and others involved in medical communication include veracity, trustworthiness, transparency, confidentiality, beneficence, nonmaleficence, autonomy, respect, justice, universalizability, and rationality.
- Ethical obligations of manuscript editors include maintaining confidentiality, avoiding favoritism, avoiding conflicts of interest or being transparent about them, avoiding and countering

overstatement, querying authors when proposing changes that might alter meaning, querying authors about conclusions that seem unsupported by evidence presented, staying current in the field, and educating authors about ethical publication practices.
- Although medical manuscript editors are not ethics police, they should be alert for indications that, perhaps inadvertently, authors are acting in ways counter to publication ethics. Some problems to be alert for are fabrication, falsification, plagiarism, duplicate publication, "salami science," inappropriate assignment of authorship, and lack of disclosure of conflicts of interest.
- If an author seems at least at risk of violating an ethical principle, sound practice can be to approach the author unconfrontationally and, if the situation appears to reflect unawareness of norms, educate the author. If it seems likely that an ethical violation does exist, the manuscript editor should inform an appropriate party, who can then decide how to proceed.

· EXERCISE ·
Cases to Consider

What are some situations in which you might apply the approaches discussed in this chapter on ethics? The following 10 cases, based on situations I have encountered or learned of, serve as examples. Included are some of the situations that seem most common. On reading these cases, you are encouraged to consider how you would approach them and why.

CASE 1: SUSPICIOUSLY SAME?

You are editing a grant proposal by a non-native user of English. In general, the prose is clear but not entirely idiomatic. However, you encounter a paragraph in which the prose is very polished. On pasting the paragraph into Google, you find that it is the same as in a published paper that the author cites. What do you think is happening here? How do you approach the situation? Why?

CASE 2: CONCEALED CONFLICTS?

You are editing a paper about a new medical device. The section where the authors should identify conflicts of interest states that none of the authors have conflicts of interest regarding the current research. However, you know that two of the authors are consultants to the company that manufactures the device. What do you think is happening here? How do you proceed? Why?

CASE 3: DÉJÀ VU?

As a manuscript editor at a medical journal, you find that an image provided as evidence in the results section of a manuscript seems strangely familiar. Upon checking, you see that it appeared in the results section of the author's previously published paper in your journal—allegedly about a different experiment. What do you think might have happened? How do you proceed? Why?

CASE 4: TOO FAST?

As an author's editor, you are reviewing a peer reviewer's report with an author and discussing how to proceed. The reviewer has said the author should do an additional experiment and add the results to the paper. However, the author protests that doing so would be too much work. Two hours later, the author returns with a version of the paper that includes the results of the requested experiment. What do you think has happened? How do you proceed? Why?

CASE 5: ABOVE AND BEYOND?

The findings of a major clinical study are about to be published in a journal. As an editor at the institution where the study was done, you are editing a news release about the findings. It appears to you that the draft of the release overstates one of the main findings of the study. Why might the seeming overstatement have occurred? How do you proceed? Why?

CASE 6: OVERLY APPRECIATIVE?

You are a member of the editorial office at a medical research institute. A large grant proposal that you edited has been accepted, and the principal investigator (PI) is thrilled. On opening a thank-you note that the PI sends you, you find that it contains a very large gift certificate to a luxury clothing store. How do you react? How do you proceed? Why?

CASE 7: WHOSE VIEWS?

You are a postdoctoral fellow hoping to pursue a medical editing career. The scientist heading the laboratory in which you work has agreed to peer-review a journal article but is very busy. Knowing your interests, the scientist asks you to do the peer review and submit it on their behalf. What do you think of the idea? How do you proceed? Why?

CASE 8: FREE ADVICE?

You are an author's editor at a health science center, and an ambitious graduate student approaches you with an idea. First, they say, they will submit the paper to the regional biomedical journal. Then, after receiving the peer reviews, they will withdraw the paper, use the peer reviews to improve it, and submit the paper to a higher-ranking journal. What do you think of the idea? How do you proceed? Why?

CASE 9: EXTRA EDITING?

You are a freelance medical editor doing some author's editing for an editing company. A manuscript seems excellent overall, and so you make few editorial changes. On receiving the edited manuscript, your contact at the editing company says you should make more changes so the authors feel they are getting their money's worth. What do you think? How do you proceed?

CASE 10: EXTRA CREDIT?

You have edited a manuscript to submit to a journal. Your editing has consisted mainly of correcting mechanical errors, increasing consistency with the journal's style, improving some of the organization, making some reasoning clearer, ensuring that references are cited where needed, and streamlining the language. The lead author is delighted with your work and offers to list you as an author. What do you think of the idea? What do you say to the lead author? Why?

· 9 ·

Careers in Medical Editing

If you've read this far in this book, or if you skipped to this chapter, you may be pursuing or seriously considering a medical editing career. What sorts of positions exist? How can you seek them? What if you're asked to take an editing test? What about certificates and certifications? If you're thinking of freelancing, what are some considerations? How can you maintain motivation during an editorial career? And what are some satisfactions of such a career? This chapter addresses such questions. So that it can be understandable on its own, the chapter overlaps somewhat with earlier material. With luck, those who have read earlier chapters will find this overlap a useful review.

Medical Editing: The Range of Substance and Settings

Medical editors may edit writing in clinical medicine, basic medical science, the medical social sciences and humanities, health policy, and more. They may edit journal articles (at any of various stages), grant proposals, regulatory documents, materials for the public, books, and—among other items—questions for examinations to license or certify health professionals. The materials edited may be destined for print or online publication, audiovisual media, or a mix. Also, medical editors may work in journal offices, universities, government agencies, health care institutions, professional associations, pharmaceutical or biotechnology companies, editing companies, freelance settings, and more. This range of substance and settings results in a wide variety of niches in medical editing. Some examples, based on editors I have known or composites thereof:

- Editor A is part of an editorial office at an institute providing specialized medical care and producing research. This editor does mainly substantive editing of manuscripts for journal submission. In addition, this editor and others in the group present sessions to educate authors. The editor also sometimes supervises editorial interns.
- Editor B is one of multiple copyeditors for a group of medical journals published by a large medical association. This editor's work consists mainly of copyediting articles accepted for publication. Other editors at this group of journals include managing editors, production editors, and web editors, as well as the journals' editors-in-chief.
- Editor C is employed by a journal published by a small medical specialty society. Because the staff is small, this editor both fulfills some functions of a managing editor and is involved in manuscript editing. This editor also is active in professional associations in science editing, thus contributing to the development of the profession.
- Editor D is a grant proposal editor at a university health science center. This editor's work entails substantively editing faculty members' proposals for external funding of research and helping to ensure that these proposals meet all requirements. This editor also helps coordinate preparation of proposals to which multiple individuals contribute.
- Editor E is in the communications group at a government agency that supports and conducts research and provides public information regarding an area of health. Among the varied items this individual edits are news releases, feature stories, fact sheets, presentations by the entity's director, blog posts, and other social media posts.
- Editor F works for a company that provides manuscript editing services to clients. The editing consists largely of editing journal submissions by international authors. Sometimes this editor also edits other materials, such as slide sets or presentation scripts for continuing education or other purposes.

- Editor G is a regulatory editor at a pharmaceutical company. This individual edits mainly materials being submitted to the government as documentation to support the approval of new drugs. Other editors at the company edit other materials, such as clinical-trial protocols, informed-consent forms, package inserts, and publications.
- Editor H works for a company that publishes books in medicine and science. As an acquisitions editor, this individual seeks potential authors for books and oversees evaluation of book proposals and manuscripts. Once a manuscript is accepted, it goes to a copyeditor—typically a freelancer with expertise in editing such content.
- Editor I is a medical features editor for an online newspaper. The work includes commissioning articles by freelance writers. Immediately beforehand, this individual, who has a medical degree and a science journalism degree, was an editor at a website for physicians. This individual moved to editorial roles after multiple years as a medical writer, mainly for online media.
- Editors J, K, and L are freelance medical editors. Editor J gradually transitioned to full-time freelance work after being an editor at a university for many years. Editor K embarked on a freelance editing career soon after completing a PhD in basic medical science. And Editor L came to freelance medical editing from a journalism career. Each edits journal submissions and some other types of writing (for example, grant proposals or textbooks).

Clearly, many niches and career paths exist in medical editing. Some medical editors remain in the same aspect of the profession throughout their careers, perhaps eventually assuming supervisory roles. Others begin in one aspect of the profession and move to another. Often, a reasonable tack is to begin where one can and then decide whether to seek a change.

In seeking a medical editing position that will suit you (and for which employers are likely to consider you well suited), several questions can be worth considering. They include the following:

- *What are your strengths?* You're most likely to break in successfully through a post that draws in part on your existing knowledge and skills. Are you trained in a health profession? Do you have a strong background in basic medical science? Do you have copyediting experience in a nonmedical field? A position that builds on such a strength is likely to be most attainable and most conducive to initial success.

- *What are your interests and values?* Do you have a passion for public health? How about clinical medicine or basic science? Does helping researchers from other countries bring you particular satisfaction? How about patient education or public outreach? Would it feel great to be part of a team that brings a new drug, device, or vaccine to market? Do you love books and dream of helping to bring them to fruition? Considering such questions can help identify niches that you would find most rewarding.
- *What sorts of working conditions suit you best?* Do you thrive most as part of a team, work most happily alone, or prefer a mix? Do a predictable routine and consistent content suit you best, or do you crave variety? Do you want clear expectations to follow, or are you comfortable (or downright happy) with ambiguity in this regard? Are you at your best under deadline pressure, or do you deteriorate under it? Do family commitments, physical limitations or health concerns, or other factors influence what would suit you best? Reflecting on such questions can aid in identifying niches that would be the happiest and most productive fit.
- *What financial considerations are there?* Do you need a well-paying position, for example because of family responsibilities or student debt? If so, a post at a major company might suit you better than one at a nonprofit. Or do you currently have no such constraints? If so, perhaps you can consider a stint working in a developing country. What about health insurance? Would employment by an institution with excellent health insurance benefits be a huge boon? Or is obtaining health insurance not a consideration, for instance because a spouse's health insurance covers you or because your country has national health insurance?
- *What geographic constraints, if any, do you have?* Traditionally, medical editing jobs have tended to cluster in locales with large medical centers, multiple medical journals, major pharmaceutical companies, or other main employers of medical editors. Thus, to work as a medical editor, one generally had to be in (or move to) one of these locales or pursue a freelance career. However, especially since the advent of the COVID-19 pandemic, opportunities for

remote employment of medical editors have become increasingly common. Therefore, although some medical editing jobs still require presence on-site, geographic constraints are less of a barrier than before. Geographic constraints can remain a consideration, though, especially for those who find working remotely less effective or less fulfilling or whose home situation is unconducive to remote work.

- *Whom would you like to work with, and in what environment?* Whether as an employee or as a freelancer, you will be interacting with others. And whether on-site or remote, you will have at least a virtual environment. Questions to consider in these regards can include the following: Do you enjoy working directly with authors, or would you prefer to have someone else be the intermediary? Do you like or loathe being in an academic environment? Are you OK with the bureaucracy encountered in academia, government, or business? Are you OK with needing to be essentially a small-business owner as a freelance editor? Do you prefer environments that are highly collaborative, or do you wish to work independently? Any other preferences regarding the workplace culture? Also, especially if you are early in your medical editing career, would the presence of mentorship be a plus for you?
- *What would you learn from the job?* Medical editing work is not only a chance to help and earn; it is also a chance to learn. Indeed, many consider the opportunity for perpetual learning a major attraction of a medical editing career. Early in your career, on-the-job learning can be important to attaining proficiency; your first job might be considered akin to a residency or fellowship. And later in your career, on-the-job learning can help maintain proficiency. Are there editorial skills you want to strengthen or editorial technologies with which you want to become more adept? Are you seeking to extend your biomedical knowledge base? Do you want work that will help keep you updated on biomedical advances? Do you favor a setting where you can partake of formal training? Would support in attending conferences be a valued perk? Such considerations too can help in deciding what sort of work to most value.

Reflecting on such questions can help in determining which opportunities to seek or prioritize. Beware, though, of holding out for what you consider perfect. Even if a position seems to entail some trade-offs, it may turn out to be—or evolve to be—one that suits you very well. And obtaining a new position once you have established yourself tends to be easier than breaking in.

Seeking and Pursuing Medical Editing Positions

Once you've identified types of medical editing positions that attract you, how can you best proceed? For example: How can you learn of openings? How can you best apply? If your application makes it through the initial screening, how can you best proceed? Many overall sources of career guidance, including university career centers, provide general advice in such regards and can be well worth consulting. The sections that follow will emphasize pointers especially applicable to seeking positions in medical editing.

IDENTIFYING OPENINGS

To identify job openings in medical editing, pursue multiple channels. Regularly search the job listing sites of organizations such as the Council of Science Editors and the American Medical Writers Association. Many societies' job sites are open only to members, but that of the Council of Science Editors, at https://councilscienceeditors-jobs.careerwebsite.com/, is open to all. Also search the job sites of specific entities, such as universities or companies, where you could envision working. If a US government job might interest you, search USAJOBS (https://www.usajobs.gov/). Likewise, if other governments (or other levels of government, such as those of states or provinces) might be potential employers, check their websites. Monitor listings on LinkedIn, which often include those for jobs in medical editing and related realms. Also look at general job websites.

In assessing whether job announcements are relevant, look at the list of duties, not only the job title. Standardized job titles for editors do not exist, and the same title sometimes refers to different types of jobs. For example, in some settings an editorial assistant is a person who performs routine copyeditorial duties. In other settings, the term is used for a person who is largely a receptionist. Similarly, the term *technical editor* has been used for a variety of roles.

Do not feel compelled to limit your search to listed jobs. For example, if working in a particular editorial office attracts you, contact the head of that office; provide information about yourself, and, if feasible, arrange an informational interview. The person will then be aware of you if jobs open up. The person also may be able to direct you to opportunities elsewhere.

While awaiting employment opportunities, keep developing your background and contacts. Participate in professional organizations; benefits can include knowing and being known when openings arise. Consider doing some volunteer editing to keep building your experience, credentials, and contacts. Let it be known throughout your professional and social circles that you are seeking a job; sometimes job leads come from unexpected sources. Also consider doing an internship (or a second or third internship) to keep building your skills, your network, and your pool of references. Perhaps do some freelance work, which can lead to employment or build credentials for it. Keep learning—about medical editing, about editing more generally, and about medical topics—through independent reading, online instruction (such as free courses through Coursera), or other means. Above all, do not sit around and mope. Staying professionally engaged, regardless of whether you have found a job, will make you a stronger candidate and prepare you to be a better employee.

The question sometimes arises of whether to apply for a position if you do not fully meet the application criteria. In general, unless a criterion (such as citizenship of a specific country) is nonnegotiable, go ahead. If the position does not come through, you will have lost nothing other than the time spent applying. And you might land the job if the dream applicant does not emerge and you are a solid candidate overall. Also, sometimes applying leads to other opportunities instead. In one such instance, the office decided to make the applicant its first intern. In another, the office kept the candidate's materials and, when a suitable opening arose, invited the candidate to apply.

COVER LETTERS

When applying for positions, you may well be asked to provide a cover letter, resume (or curriculum vitae), and list of references. All three can be chances to showcase relevant abilities through skillful writing and sound formatting. Of course, they should be thoroughly proofread.

The cover letter should be geared to the specific opportunity rather than being a form letter. It should contain keywords from the job description, both to help your application pass any initial screening by AI bots or human resource staff and so search committee members or potential supervisors can readily discern your match with the position. It generally should not exceed about one page, and it normally should have three main parts. The first part should be a brief paragraph identifying the opening being applied for and, if appropriate, providing brief context. Some examples:

- "I am pleased to apply for the newly announced medical editor position at the XYZ Institute."
- "As a recent recipient of a master's degree in science writing and editing, I am pleased to apply for the newly announced medical editor position at the XYZ Institute."
- "As a recent recipient of a master's degree in science writing and editing, I am pleased to apply for the newly announced medical editor position at the XYZ Institute. Dr. Barbara Gastel, who directs our master's program, recommended that I apply."

If the job announcement lists an identification number for the position, the opening paragraph should include that number.

The next section should summarize your qualifications for the position as described in the job announcement (and, if applicable, as ascertained through other means, such as online research about the employer). This section should present highlights of your resume or CV and put them in context by telling your story. Like much good writing, it should show rather than tell; for example, rather than using the terms *hardworking*, *knowledgeable*, *collaborative*, and *helpful*, it should present evidence from which readers can surmise that you have these attributes. The following are three fictional examples. The first two are from early-career applicants. The third is from someone more senior who seeks to transition to an editorial position.

- "I have long been interested in both communication and science. As an undergraduate at ___ University, I majored in English and minored in biology. I was science editor of our college newspaper and a student writer in our veterinary school communications office. I then completed the master's degree program in science journalism at ___ University. In addition to courses in science editing and science writing, I took graduate courses in several areas of biomedical science, including epidemiology, physiology, and pharmacology. I also completed an editorial internship at ___ Clinic. During graduate school I was a teaching assistant for a course in biomedical writing and a writing consultant at our university writing center. I was therefore pleased to see that the position I am seeking includes not only editing manuscripts but also helping to give workshops on writing."

- "A neuroscientist by training, I have come to realize that my interests and strengths lie mainly in communicating science rather than doing research myself. In college, I enjoyed serving as manuscript editor of my university's student science journal. During my doctoral studies, my favorite activities have been writing proposals and journal articles, and others in my department have often called on me to help edit their work. I also prefer continually learning about varied research rather than investigating a narrow topic. A graduate course in science editing introduced me to editorial careers, and participating in the regional chapter of the American Medical Writers Association has confirmed that medical editing is a field for me. My strong biomedical background will, I believe, be an asset in the position I am seeking, and the prospect of receiving mentorship as a junior member of your team especially appeals to me."
- "My professional focus has been moving increasingly to medical editing. After receiving a journalism degree from ABC University, I began my career as a general reporter. I then served as health reporter for the *DEF Tribune* for six years, until cutbacks resulted in the closing of the health and science desk. Afterward, I spent two years as a magazine copyeditor. I have been freelancing full-time for the past five years; whereas initially my freelance work consisted mainly of writing health articles, it now consists largely of editing such articles for clients. Meanwhile, as listed in my resume, I have continued strengthening my medical editing background by taking courses and participating in professional organizations. Given my background, I feel well suited for the associate medical editor position in the marketing and communications office of GHI Medical Center, and I believe that the position would be an exciting next step in my career."

The last part of the letter should be a brief paragraph summing up and encouraging positive action. Some possibilities:

- "Thank you for your attention. I believe that this position is a fine match with my background and goals, and I hope to be granted the opportunity to explore it further."
- "Thank you for your attention. I would value the opportunity to work as a medical editor at ____, and I would be honored to receive an interview."

This ending should sound confident (not desperate!). However, it should not sound arrogant; a statement such as "I look forward to working with you" may elicit a reaction such as "You might look forward to it, but you're not going to do so."

PREPARING RESUMES AND LISTING REFERENCES

For corporate positions, a resume is likely to be requested. For academic positions, a curriculum vitae (commonly called a CV) may be requested instead. The two tend to be much the same for early-career applicants. For applicants later in their careers, the two diverge. For example, resumes tend to be limited to a page or two regardless of career stage, whereas CVs can run several pages or more. Resumes are more likely than CVs to contain bulleted lists of job duties; CVs are more likely than resumes to have detailed lists of publications. Regardless of whether you will provide a resume or a CV, the following pointers can help when applying for medical editing posts:

- Keep the design simple and straightforward. Also make it conducive to skimming, for instance by using boldface for major items. Edit for conciseness and readability. Include ample white space.
- In the heading, include contact information that will remain valid. For example, if you're a student, provide a long-term email address rather than your school one. Also ensure that your email address sounds professional; for example, *bjgastel@gmail.com* is suitable, whereas *barb-likes-baking@gmail.com* conveys the impression that the person's priorities lie elsewhere. Try to make sure as well that your email address sounds contemporary; a Hotmail or Yahoo! address may suggest that you are behind the times.
- As in the cover letter, show rather than tell. Rather than using adjectives to describe your traits, list items that show you have

them. Your education, job history, honors, and other entries all can demonstrate that you have qualities being sought.

- Prominently feature items directly applicable to medical editing (or to the aspect of it in which you wish to work). Examples include relevant degrees, certificates, and certifications; completion of coursework in the field; proficiencies with relevant styles (such as AMA, APA, and CSE); and memberships in relevant professional societies (such as the American Medical Writers Association, the Council of Science Editors, and the European Association of Science Editors).
- You need not list every experience. On the other hand, do not feel limited to including experiences directly related to the work you seek. Listing other experiences—for example in other service roles—also can show that you have applicable knowledge, skills, and traits. If you have several transferable experiences of the same type, consider grouping them as a single entry rather than taking the space to list each. For example, you might be able to say "Teaching assistant for undergraduate biology courses," "Physical therapist at rehabilitation facilities," or "Counselor at summer science camps."
- Similarly, if you are just embarking on your career and have some experiences too small to merit individual listing, consider grouping them. (Example: "Editing and proofreading poster presentations, application essays, and other materials for fellow students.")
- Consider adapting your resume or CV to the position sought or having different versions for different types of work (for example, copyediting versus author's editing). For instance, if you have taken courses especially relevant to a given job, perhaps list them. Or if the position has an instructional component, maybe include more than otherwise about your experience teaching, tutoring, or mentoring. Likewise, you can reorganize your resume or CV such that the parts most relevant to a position come earlier in it. If a resume or CV is for a specific position, try to ensure that it contains keywords from the job announcement, especially if the position is at a large entity where applications may be screened by AI bots or by staff unversed in medical editing.
- Ensure that your resume or CV evidences your editorial astuteness. Of course, proofread it carefully. Make sure, for example, that consistency exists in conventions followed for punctuation; that lists show good parallelism; and that bibliographic entries (if any) are

formatted consistently. You might especially impress those hiring if the editorial office follows a specific style and your resume or CV is in that style; for instance, when applying to work at a journal that uses AMA style, a resume or CV that complies with AMA style is likely to be a plus.

When submitting a job application or later in the application process, you may be asked to list *professional references*—in other words, people who know your work and can vouch for your abilities and attributes. Those hiring may then consult these individuals, especially if you are a finalist for the position. Applicants who are established in their fields commonly include former supervisors as references. If, however, you are early in your career or transitioning to medical editing, you might not have medical editing employers to list. In such cases, appropriate references may include people such as the following: faculty members well acquainted with your work as a student, advisors of extracurricular activities in which you have had major roles, internship supervisors, and supervisors in jobs requiring some of the skills and traits needed in medical editing. Freelance clients also can be appropriate to list. Because professional references, not character references, are being sought, generally do not list people such as friends or clergy unless they know you in a professional capacity (such as editing the congregation's newsletter). Before listing people, obtain their permission. Also, if it seems likely that they will indeed be contacted (for example, because you become a finalist for a position), alert them and provide background, such as the job description and your current resume or CV, so they can be prepared.

Just as you can have different versions of your resume or CV to suit different positions, you can list different references depending on the position being applied for. Regardless of who is included, the list of references should reflect your editorial skill. For example, all content should be checked for accuracy, and items such as degrees and contact information should be in a consistent format. Also, follow up with the individuals listed. Especially if you receive a job for which they have served as references, let them know, and convey your thanks.

INTERVIEWING AND BEYOND

If you are being seriously considered for a position, you probably will receive one or more interviews for it. These interviews may be in person, or they may be online—for instance, via a platform such as Zoom or Microsoft Teams. The interviews may be one-on-one, or two or more people may interview you at once. A few basic tips:

- *Research the entity at which you would be working.* For example, if the job is at a medical journal, become familiar with the journal and its instructions to authors. Or if the job is at a medical research institution, look carefully at its website, noticing items such as types of research done and values conveyed. Becoming informed can help both in answering questions suitably and in formulating questions of your own.
- *If the interview will be online, prepare accordingly.* Be familiar with the platform. Arrange for the interview to be in a quiet place, without interruptions from household members or pets. Be mindful of the background; if your environment looks unprofessional or otherwise unsuitable, opt for a tasteful virtual background or set the platform to blur the background. Dress as you would for an interview in person. So that people can readily see you (rather than just a silhouette of your head), have light shining on your face, either from a lamp or from a window. Make sure your computer's camera is at a suitable height relative to your face, so viewers aren't looking at the top of your head or up your nose. Arrive early, in case of technical difficulties. And if technical difficulties do arise, keep your cool.
- *Answer what is asked.* Develop answers well, but stay focused. Answer truthfully, rather than striving always to say what you imagine the interviewer wants to hear. Keep in mind points you hope to convey in the interview, in case chances arise to bridge to them from other discussion and in case you are asked whether you wish to add anything.
- *Do not feel compelled to answer each question instantly.* Feel free to take a little time to think. A thoughtful, deliberate approach is likely to be appreciated in a medical editor.
- *If you don't know the answer to a question, say so.* Perhaps say how you would seek the answer. Likewise, if you lack a skill that is being asked about, say so, without being defensive; perhaps explain how you could go about obtaining the skill and note previous success in gaining such skills.
- *Display qualities likely to be sought.* For example: Be punctual. Be articulate, while realizing that spoken language is not as polished

as written language. Be attentive. In what you say and how you say it, avoid anything that may suggest that you lack tact or empathy or judgment. If you discuss an unfavorable experience, avoid griping; rather, frame the experience positively, for example in terms of insights gained.

- *Have questions ready.* As well as letting you learn more about the job and its context, doing so shows that you are interested and engaged. In initial interviews, the questions should focus largely on the work. They may also address related topics, such as opportunities for continued learning. During initial interviews, generally avoid asking about subjects such as salary and vacation time; such questions typically belong later, once the entity has offered you a job or has let you know that it wishes to do so.
- *Show enthusiasm.* Display interest in the job and the interviewer(s). Such enthusiasm tends to be contagious. It also helps show that you would be an active, committed employee.
- *Realize that the interview is a two-way process.* Not only are the interviewers evaluating your fit for the job; the interview can also help you consider whether the job fits from your standpoint. From what you learned in the interview, does the nature of the work indeed seem to suit you? From what you have observed of your interviewers—and, if seen, their interactions—do you envision liking the work environment? Does the culture of the journal, company, or other entity appeal to you? If your interview was on-site, what about the physical environment? Reflecting on such questions can help you decide whether to accept the job if offered.

So, the interview phase has gone well, your references have spoken highly of you, and you are being offered the job! Should you accept it? Among factors to consider are the work; the salary; other benefits such as health insurance and retirement funds; the colleagues; opportunities for professional advancement; opportunities for continued learning; whether the work is on-site, remote, or hybrid (and for each of these, the working circumstances); and policies of personal relevance to you (perhaps, for example, those regarding parental leave or flexible working hours). If, based on such factors, the opportunity seems promising overall, discussing the terms of acceptance can follow. For some positions, opportunity to negotiate about salaries exists; for others, salary criteria are strictly set. Even if the entering salary cannot be increased, an employer sometimes can offer other pluses, such as covering some translocation costs (if you would need to move to the employer's locale) or paying for annual travel to a professional conference.

Reflect on the full picture in terms of both what you are seeking now and how the position could relate to further developing your medical editing career. Also consider your intuition about the offer; does the position excite you, or do you have nagging doubts? Perhaps discuss the decision with family members, friends, mentors, or others who know you well and whose judgment you value. A perfect position might not exist, but if you find one that can help you break into medical editing (or enter the next phase of your medical editing career), go with it—and don't look back. Approach the job with enthusiasm and energy, and strive to make it a fine experience and to excel in your medical editing position. You are then likely to progress well in your medical editing career.

Taking Medical Editing Tests for Employment

Evaluating candidates for medical editing opportunities sometimes includes testing their medical editing skill. Individuals being considered for staff or freelance employment may therefore be asked to take medical editing tests. The tests are of two main types. In one type, candidates receive a set of short items, such as sentences or paragraphs, to edit. In the other, candidates receive a manuscript to edit, and the editing is evaluated. Some of the tests are timed tests under supervision; others are take-home tests to be submitted by a deadline. Research (Boettger 2012) has identified some types of errors commonly included in medical editing tests from a sample of medical communication companies.

Drawing largely on a classic article presenting advice on the subject (Whalen 1992), 10 tips for taking editing tests for employment are as follows:

1. Read, and follow, the instructions carefully. Your ability to comply with instructions may be among items being assessed.
2. If it is not specified, find out what resources, if any, you can consult during the test.
3. If you are allowed to consult whatever resources you wish, ask what style manual to use. As well as helping with the test, doing so may show your awareness of such considerations.
4. Realize that perfection is not expected on such tests. Just do your best.

5. If the test is timed, pace yourself. If it is untimed, consider asking how much time typically is expected. In any case, devote just a reasonable amount of time to the test. There is no point in setting an expectation that you cannot achieve under normal conditions.
6. If the test includes querying, compose queries skillfully. In particular, try to ensure that they are clear, concise, and courteous. Of course, make sure that the queries do not have mechanical errors. Avoid over-querying.
7. If the test occasionally contains items that you would check but that you lack the time or resources to check, perhaps briefly note how you would check them.
8. Try to avoid overediting. Remember that introducing an error tends to be worse than leaving an error uncorrected. And remember that you are editing, not rewriting.
9. Recognize the test as a way to also assess the potential employer. If the test seems unreasonable or emphasizes tasks that don't suit you, perhaps question whether the work being sought is a suitable match. Or if the test is reasonable, well administered, and perhaps even enjoyable, take it as a sign that the opportunity may be a good fit.
10. Of course, submit the completed test on time. Also show professionalism in other regards when interacting with those administering such tests. For example, show a positive attitude, communicate adeptly, and express appreciation for the opportunity to be considered.

It has been at least rumored that unscrupulous employers have used the latter type of editing test, where the candidate edits an entire manuscript, to obtain free editing. If employers will use work done on editing tests as a professional product rather than only evaluating it, they should pay the test-takers for the work, regardless of whether the test-takers end up being hired. If for an editing test you are asked to do editing that takes many hours, ask about being compensated.

Certificates and Certifications

Unlike medical editing tests, which generally are from individual employers, certificates and certifications more generally document background or demonstrate proficiency. The terms *certificate* and *certification* sometimes are mistakenly interchanged. However, certificates and certifications differ from each other. A certificate attests to having successfully completed a set of educational activities. It indicates effective exposure but not necessarily broader proficiency. In contrast, a certification attests to at least basic proficiency. Obtaining a certification generally requires having at least a specified amount of experience in the field and passing a rigorous comprehensive examination. Certifications tend to remain valid for a limited number of years. Commonly, they can be renewed by retaking the examination or documenting adequate continuing education or the equivalent. Certificates and certifications help demonstrate to employers or clients a medical editor's commitment, knowledge, and ability. They also can contribute to a medical editor's self-confidence.

Certificates for medical editors have tended to be in the combined fields of medical writing and editing. At least in the United States, the most prominent such certificates are those from the American Medical Writers Association (AMWA) and from certificate programs associated with universities. The AMWA Essential Skills certificate program (https://www.amwa.org/general/custom.asp?page=ES_Certificate) entails completing seven self-study modules and passing the final exam in each. Two leading university-associated certificate programs are the University of Chicago certificate program in medical writing and editing (https://professional.uchicago.edu/find-your-fit/certificates/medical-writing-and-editing) and the University of California, San Diego, medical writing certificate program (https://extendedstudies.ucsd.edu/courses-and-programs/medical-writing-courses). Both programs are online. The former entails completing six online courses, including a course in medical copyediting and one in substantive editing; the latter includes combined courses in medical writing and editing. These certificate programs are for college graduates; many registrants also have graduate or professional degrees. Registrants range from recent college graduates seeking to enter the field, to mid-career individuals wanting to strengthen their medical editing work or transition to such work, to retirees thinking of pursuing medical editing.

More recently, AMWA has established a certificate specifically in medical editing (https://amwa.mycrowdwisdom.com/cw/course-details?entryId=14219083&subscribed=false). Obtaining this certificate entails completing 11 online activities, most or all of which already were available individually, and completing a "knowledge check" after each. As well as some basics of copyediting and proofreading, topics of the activities include such items as querying authors, working with authors who are non-native users of English, editing for conciseness, and "removing nonempathetic language." An activity on tables and graphs also is included. The stated total completion time for the set of activities is 8.5 hours. Thus, this certificate program seems less extensive than the AMWA Essential Skills program and the university-associated certificate programs noted above. Employers hiring medical editors may be aware that different professional certificates earned by medical editors can reflect different scopes of instruction.

In contrast to certificates, certifications focus on proficiency shown rather than instruction completed. For medical editors (and other editors in biologically related fields), a well-recognized credential in this regard is certification by the Board of Editors in the Life Sciences (https://www.bels.org/), commonly known as BELS, which was established in 1991. To be eligible for BELS certification, individuals generally need at least a bachelor's degree and two years' manuscript editing experience in the life sciences, such as medical science. Obtaining BELS certification requires passing a rigorous examination. The examination, which is given via computer, can be taken at testing locations in more than 160 countries; it also can be taken at home or in another remote location. The BELS certification study guide (https://www.bels.org/study-guide)—which provides information about the examination and its administration and includes sample questions—lists (in alphabetical order) the following as the topics tested: bibliographic references; grammar; internal consistency; mechanics; numbers; organization; publishing requirements; punctuation; syntax; tables and illustrations; traditional principles and ethics of scientific inquiry, writing, and publishing; units of measure and scientific terms; and usage and diction. Individuals with BELS certification can place the initials "ELS" after their names. BELS certification is valid for five years. Certification can be renewed either by retaking and passing the BELS examination or by earning credits for activities in professional development or related realms. Among activities that can earn credits are attending or giving presentations or courses, obtaining or providing mentorship, providing service to relevant professional organizations, and writing articles in the field.

Another certification for medical editors to consider seeking is the Medical Writer Certified (MWC) credential (https://www.amwa.org/page/MWC), obtained through the American Medical Writers Association (AMWA). Unlike BELS certification, the MWC credential is specifically medical. And although it has only "medical writer" in its title, the proficiencies that it reflects also apply to medical editing. Like BELS certification, obtaining the MWC credential requires passing a computer-based examination that is offered at multiple locations worldwide. Eligibility criteria for taking the examination include having at least a bachelor's degree and two years' paid work experience in medical communication. A study guide from AMWA (https://cdn.ymaws.com/www.amwa.org/resource/resmgr/certification/forms/2024/MWCStudyGuideResourceList2-2.pdf) describes the scope of the examination, provides sample questions, and identifies resources that can aid in preparing for the examination. To keep the MWC credential, recipients must recertify every five years. One way to do so is by successfully retaking the MWC examination; the other is by earning enough points for continuing-education activities or related endeavors in areas related to the examination content.

A third certification that medical editors can seek is the Certified Medical Publication Professional (CMPP) credential, from the International Society for Medical Publication Professionals (ISMPP). This organization, formed in 2005, emphasizes "the ethical and effective communication of medical research to inform treatment decisions" (https://www.ismpp.org/) and tends to have a corporate emphasis. To obtain the CMPP credential, candidates must have a sufficient mix of education and experience and pass a computerized examination largely on publication planning. Certification is valid for five years, after which recertification can be obtained by successfully retaking the examination or by earning a requisite number of continuing-education credits. Information on the CMPP certification appears at https://www.ismpp.org/certification.

Considerations for Freelance Medical Editors

Many medical editors freelance, either as their main employment or in addition to holding full- or part-time positions. Such work can be both literally and figuratively rewarding. However, it also can pose pitfalls. Attentiveness to several considerations can help maximize the rewards and minimize the risks. This section touches on some such considerations. Resources for exploring such considerations more extensively include materials from the Editorial Freelancers Association (https://www.the-efa.org/), items available on or through the American Medical Writers

Association website, and *The Chicago Guide for Freelance Editors: How to Take Care of Your Business, Your Clients, and Yourself from Start-Up to Sustainability* (Brenner 2024).

A basic question is why you are considering freelance work. If you hope to freelance in addition to your existing employment: Do you mainly want extra income? Are you hoping that the freelancing will lead to a medical editing position? Are you wanting to transition to full-time freelancing? Are you seeking intellectual stimulation? Are you largely wanting to serve those unable to otherwise afford such assistance? Something else? Some combination? The answer might help determine whether, for example, you seek mainly to freelance for corporate clients or to assist authors from low- and middle-income countries. It may also influence other aspects of your approach.

If you freelance on the side, also keep the following in mind. Of course, avoid conflicts of interest. For example, you should not freelance for your employer's competitor. And avoid conflicts of commitment; it is unfair to stay up all night doing a freelance project and then come to work too exhausted to concentrate. Some employers require that outside work be approved in advance; remember to file the needed paperwork. Also, remember that even if you consider your freelancing a hobby, the government does not. So, be sure to record and report your freelance income and to pay the needed taxes (including, if required, quarterly estimated taxes).

If you are thinking of freelancing full-time, likewise consider your motivations and their implications. For example: Do you want to freelance so you can focus on your favorite type of work? Are you freelancing because you want to do varied work? Do you want to freelance mainly so you can be your own boss or so you can work at home? Is your priority to choose how much work you do and when you do it? Are you freelancing because of geographic constraints? Are you doing so because you lost your job or have yet to find one? Something else? Some mix of the above? Again, the answer may influence your approach.

A major consideration in whether (and if so, how) to freelance as your sole employment is how much income you need or want. If, for example, you are a recent graduate without other financial resources, it may be wise to defer freelancing until you amass some savings, pay off any student debt, and gain more professional experience and contacts. (Especially at the beginning, freelance income can be unpredictable. Therefore, it generally is wise to have several months' living expenses saved before embarking on freelancing full-time.) You may have much more freedom about when to start freelancing full-time, and what freelance work to do, if you need not depend on current freelance earnings—for example, because you have a spouse or partner with adequate income for the household, are pursuing a freelance career after retirement, or are independently wealthy (a rarity for medical editors).

A gradual transition to full-time freelancing often works well. For example, medical editors sometimes cut back to part-time work for their longtime employers while making the transition. Often, those employers become major clients once the transition is complete. Also, especially during the transition, willingness to do some work other than medical editing per se can be helpful. For example, medical editors can complement their medical editing income with income from nonmedical editing or from medical writing.

Prospective freelancers may dream of focusing on medical manuscripts throughout their working hours. However, a freelancer is the runner of a small business. Thus, succeeding as a freelancer requires devoting time and attention to the business aspects. Indeed, the decision whether to freelance may depend in part on whether one likes, or at least can tolerate, those aspects. Common such aspects include setting up an office (either in your home or in rented space), establishing and maintaining a website, ensuring availability of adequate information technology (IT) support, making sure to have suitable insurance relating to your work, marketing your services (often less of a consideration later, once you have established clients and solid sources of referrals), dealing with contracts, managing workflow, keeping track of hours, billing clients, paying for health insurance if you are not otherwise covered, paying taxes, saving for retirement, paying subcontractors and such, and finding and paying professionals such as accountants and lawyers.

One issue that freelancers face is deciding what rates to charge (or determining which projects with set rates pay enough to consider). One resource in this regard is *What to Charge: Pricing Strategies for Freelancers and Consultants*, by Laurie Lewis (Lewis 2011). Another resource is the editorial rate chart (https://www.the-efa.org/rates/) on the Editorial Freelancers Association (EFA) website. The rates in this chart may be somewhat low, especially for very experienced medical editors, but they provide some perspective. Further perspective can be gained from reports on the medical communication compensation surveys conducted every few years by the American Medical Writers Association (AMWA).

As noted, the EFA, AMWA, and other groups also are resources more broadly for freelancing. For example, the EFA website has an extensive section titled "Resources for New Freelance Editors," and the AMWA website includes a large section, "Expert Tips for Freelance Medical Writing," containing much that addresses or applies to medical editing as well. The website of ACES: The Society for Editing also has materials on freelancing, and the website of *Science Editor* (the periodical of the Council of Science Editors) includes freelancing-related articles from the publication. Also, the EFA has a member directory, the AMWA website includes a directory of freelancers, and the BELS website contains a directory of BELS-certified editors who freelance; all three directories are openly available. Other resources include venues such as the EFA email discussion list and the AMWA online community AMWA Engage. The archives of such discussion venues contain a wealth of information on everything from choosing an office chair to addressing ethical issues. And monitoring and contributing to the discussions can be a fine way to keep up on editorial topics and more generally be part of the editorial community.

Speaking of community: Freelance medical editing can be professionally isolating, as can employment as the only medical editor in a setting. But especially given current technology, physical separation from other medical editors need not spell isolation. Discussion lists and other online forums, video meetings through applications such as Zoom, online conferences, and email and phone and chat enable ready interaction with other medical editors regardless of location. Take advantage of such opportunities. Also, to get to know other medical editors, consider volunteering for a committee of a relevant organization. If feasible, physically attend some meetings of such organizations or their chapters, if any. Through organizations or otherwise, seek medical editing mentors. And as your career progresses, be available as a mentor. In such ways, you can become not only a medical editor but also part of the medical editing community. Both your work and your spirit are likely to benefit.

Working Remotely

Whether across town or across the world, you almost certainly work remotely if you freelance. Increasingly, medical editors with staff positions also work remotely at least part of the time. Of course, different editors working remotely have different contexts, preferences, resources, and constraints. The following, though, are suggestions to consider for working productively, efficiently, and comfortably when remote.

- *Choose or establish a workspace conducive to your working style.* For some aspects to consider, see the section "Tools for Your Office" in chapter 2.
- *Consider how to dress.* For some of us, benefits of remote work include the ability to work in sweats or pajamas (except during video calls). Others of us feel more professional and tend to be more productive if dressed more formally, though still comfortably.
- *Consider your working hours.* Flexibility in when to work can be a plus of remote work. If you have a staff position, though, you may need to work standard business hours or at least during core hours. Even if you have no such requirements, consider what schedule would work best. Considerations may include whether you tend to be most productive with a regular routine, what times of day you have other demands, what times you tend to work best, and what times authors and others with whom you must communicate are available.
- Of course, *make good use of communication technologies*. Email, messaging apps, and videoconferencing all can aid in being effectively connected. Be proactive in using them. And don't neglect the telephone. Also, consider the preferences of authors and others with whom you communicate—and their responsiveness to various channels.
- *If you are joining an editorial office as a remote member, perhaps request an "onboarding buddy"* (Jakubisin 2023)—in other words, a more experienced team member who can help orient you, answer your questions, and make you feel included. If you head an editorial office, consider assigning onboarding buddies to new remote hires.
- To help ensure that you stay connected, *perhaps incorporate communication routines*. For example, have regularly scheduled online meetings with the rest of your team, with your supervisor or supervisee or intern, or with collaborators on a project. Maybe have particular times of day to check email.
- To avoid burnout, *remember to take breaks*. Maybe incorporate some exercise into your breaks. Rest your eyes. Maybe go outside. Try to avoid heading to the refrigerator during every break.
- *Maintain enough human contact*. Different editors working remotely have different amounts of human contact outside of work. And

different ones want different amounts. But avoid the risk of social isolation. Perhaps make a point of going to lunch from time to time with a friend or colleague. Maybe do some in-person volunteer work. Perhaps become active in a local organization. One way or another, be with others.

- *Become, or remain, part of the medical editing community.* As discussed at the end of the section on freelancing, participate in this community through professional organizations and in other ways. Thus, continue learning from other medical editors and contributing to their learning.

Sources of guidance on working fully or partly remote include an article by a Council of Science Editors member with longtime experience in these regards (Landis 2023). This article includes tips for working from home (as remote workers generally do): setting boundaries (regarding where and when you work, and regarding interruptions from others in the household), practicing good meeting etiquette (such as minimizing background distractions and avoiding multitasking), taking the initiative to connect personally with colleagues, and making yourself visible. Other tips for working remotely can readily be found on the internet.

Continuing to Develop as a Medical Editor

Both medicine and editing are continually changing fields. Therefore, medical editors need to keep up.

It is not necessary—and, indeed, is not possible—to keep up with everything in medicine. Rather, a reasonable approach for an editor tends to have two aspects: learning new specifics as the need arises, and staying medically informed overall, so you maintain a sound framework. Learning specifics as need arises in your work may include initially reading lay materials to orient yourself and then reading journal articles or other technical materials. It may also include being briefed by authors or other experts, including fellow editors. And it may include accessing presentations online. Staying medically informed overall generally entails at least staying up with medical news through major media and reading medical feature stories in newspapers or magazines or elsewhere. It may also include attending presentations or webinars. And, especially if you do relatively technical medical editing, it may include at least browsing through general medical journals or journals focusing on the medical subject areas in which you edit.

Many resources can help us keep up in editing—and specifically in medical editing. Perhaps chief among them are professional organizations such as the Council of Science Editors, the European Association of Science Editors, and the American Medical Writers Association. Such organizations' publications, conferences, webinars, email discussion lists, online forums, and other offerings are prime resources for keeping up—and for learning of other resources for keeping up. Informal interactions with editorial colleagues also can aid in keeping current. So can online instruction, including that available through many institutions where medical editors work.

When this book was being written, a field moving especially fast was artificial intelligence (AI), including its use in medical communication. So much was changing that clearly anything definitive in this regard would be out of date before the book even saw print. Throughout, though, resources such as those noted in the paragraph above were useful in keeping up—and in identifying specialized resources such as the blog AI Sidequest: How-To Tips and News (https://ai-sidequest.beehiiv.com/) from Mignon Fogarty, perhaps better known as Grammar Girl. Regardless of how AI continues to develop, a strong foundation in the basics of medical editing—as I hope the current book provides—is likely to be crucial in knowing when and how to use it in medical editing and how to evaluate and refine its output. Likewise, such a foundation can readily be built on more generally as technology, society, and one's own interests continue to evolve.

Notably, many careers in medical editing entail more than medical editing per se. For example, they may include teaching, project management, or people management. Or they may benefit from some understanding of statistical methods or graphic design. Courses or self-study in such areas can help a medical editor keep up—and move up.

Maintaining Motivation

Medical editing can be intense and often solitary work. Thus, medical editors risk burnout. Yet ways exist to help maintain motivation. The following are some to consider.

In keeping with the previous section, *network with peers* through professional organizations or otherwise. Commiserate about frustrations. Brainstorm about solutions. Trade tips. Share successes. Come away re-energized. Also *cultivate other contacts and other interests.* As immersive as medical editing can be, spend some time with people in other fields. And despite the press of deadlines, take some time for other pursuits. After talking with your neighbor the musician, cooking a meal, or playing your favorite sport, you may return refreshed.

Continue expanding and updating your editorial and medical knowledge. Editing and medicine keep evolving. When medical editors now in their late careers entered the field, editing was done solely on paper, electronic journals did not exist, and AI was a figment of fiction. Computed tomographic (CT) scans were first becoming available, use of the polymerase chain reaction (PCR) had not yet become a major laboratory technique, and AIDS and COVID-19 had not yet emerged. Even at a given time, editorial knowledge and medical knowledge are nearly boundless. Today, medical editors can keep learning both through traditional means such as articles, books, and face-to-face courses and through webinars, podcasts, massive open online courses (MOOCs), and more. As well as enhancing your ability as a medical editor, taking advantage of opportunities to keep learning can help maintain your enthusiasm.

Consider varying your work. To help stay fresh and maintain motivation, maybe vary your work, either by including additional areas of medical editing or by becoming involved in related realms. For instance, if you have been editing journal articles, maybe edit an article for general readers or a book chapter. Perhaps do some volunteer editing for Rising Scholars (https://risingscholars.net/en/) or for a medical or other organization whose mission you value. Or volunteer to judge entries for writing awards such as those from the National Association of Science Writers or the Association of Health Care Journalists. Perhaps do some writing yourself, venture into other media, or do some teaching. Such variety can expand your horizons and help sustain your motivation.

Take breaks. Whether under deadline pressure or just immersed in the work, you may find yourself editing for hours at a time day after day. Take breaks, though, to rest your eyes and your mind. Perhaps build some breaks into your calendar—for example, by scheduling lunches with colleagues or friends or by having set times to exercise. Your editing and your attitude are likely to be better for it. And yes, *get exercise.* Editing tends to be sedentary. Find types of exercise that suit your personality, tastes, and circumstances, and make time to exercise. Your health and your concentration are likely to benefit.

Eschew perfectionism. Medical editors should indeed have high standards. Important content is at stake, and readers, authors, and publishers deserve your best effort. However, perfection is unreasonable to expect. Even the most skilled and careful copyeditors occasionally miss items. And in substantive editing, some problems are subtle or lack ideal solutions. Do not let the occasional imperfection erode your self-confidence, squelch your enjoyment of medical editing, or sap your motivation. Rather, when you notice that absence of a serial comma, that number that should have been a numeral, or that passage that would have benefited from reorganization, think how you could avoid missing such items in the future, and move on.

Appreciate the humor. As a medical editor, you'll doubtless come across bloopers that are howlers. Some I've encountered: *amphibious* for *ambidextrous, bone degeneracy* for *bone degeneration, centurions* for *centenarians, host spices* for *host species, hypocritic oath* for *Hippocratic oath, lumber puncture* for *lumbar puncture, regiment* for *regimen, warm the public about risks* for *warn the public about risks*, and *wildly available* for *widely available*. I've also encountered *accusation editor* for *acquisitions editor, adjutant professor* for *adjunct professor, compressive exam* for *comprehensive exam, edible file* for *editable file, entomology of difficult words* for *etymology of difficult words, illicit* for *elicit, pier-reviewed publications* for *peer-reviewed publications, pneumonic* for *mnemonic, redaction* for *retraction, sanskrit fonts* for *sans serif fonts, the most impotent findings* for *the most important findings, upmost* for *utmost*, and *viscous cycle* for *vicious cycle*. One medical trainee wrote of what *perspired* (presumably *transpired*) during a patient's hospitalization, and another wrote that surgery *exasperated* (presumably *exacerbated*) a patient's weakness. And then there's the sentence "It also provides advice on how to prevent injuries from sports medicine physicians." (Presumably the advice, not the injuries, came from the physicians.) Enjoy such items when you encounter them. And, in keeping with distinguished precedent (Loviglio 1999, also a source of more such examples), perhaps keep a file of such items, and take it out when the going gets rough. Some good laughs can defuse tension and maintain motivation.

Take stock of your impact and successes. Although focusing on problems is integral to the editorial mindset, remember to notice your impact and successes as a medical editor. Think of the authors you have helped publish a paper, win a grant, or convey their message better to practitioners, researchers, or general readers. Consider audiences who have benefited from your making medical writing clearer, more polished, and otherwise sounder. If applicable, note the publishers, institutions, or other entities whose standards you have helped meet and whose goals you have helped promote through your work. Remember that ultimately your work is helping to advance medicine and promote health. Also keep track of praise. When grateful authors send you notes of appreciation, keep copies in a file. Ditto for praise from supervisors and others. Look at the file on days that nothing seems to go right and you are wondering whether to continue. Knowing that as a medical editor you are making valuable contributions can help maintain your motivation.

Satisfactions of Medical Editing

In keeping with points at the end of the previous section, medical editing can bring many satisfactions (Gastel 2011). It is a challenging, intellectually stimulating craft that can generate the joy of solving puzzles. It has an aesthetic element as well, and so it can yield the satisfaction of helping to create a well-crafted product. It provides the opportunity, and often the need, to continually learn—about medicine, about editing, and more. It often includes interaction and collaboration with bright, interesting, engaged people, including medical authors, fellow medical editors, and others on publication teams. It also offers the satisfaction of aiding authors, publishers, readers, and ultimately patients through what is essentially a helping profession.

I hope this book has conveyed these satisfactions—and has helped you to cultivate the craft of medical editing and explore possibilities for medical editing careers. Whether you embark on a medical editing career, use this book to enhance your current medical editing career, or apply the content in other ways, I wish you much satisfaction and success.

Key Points

- Medical editors may edit any of a wide variety of materials. They also work in a wide variety of settings.
- Aspects to consider in deciding which medical editing opportunities to seek include one's strengths, interests, values, preferred working conditions, financial situation, geographic constraints, and

preferences regarding colleagues, working environment, and learning opportunities.

- Ways to identify job openings in medical editing include professional organizations, job websites of potential employers, and more general employment websites. Even if a job has not been announced, reaching out to a desired employer can be fruitful.
- Each cover letter should be geared specifically to the position being applied for. Likewise, resumes and CVs can be adapted to the position being sought.
- In interviews, displaying qualities that befit a medical editor is useful. Also, an interview is a two-way process and thus a chance to evaluate the potential employer.
- Those being considered for medical editing jobs may be given medical editing tests. Some of these tests are short-answer. Others entail editing a piece of medical writing.
- Various certificates and certifications exist in areas that include medical editing. These certificates and certifications can attest to a medical editor's knowledge, skill, and commitment.
- Among considerations for freelance medical editors are the reasons freelancing was chosen (and thus the approach to take), the amount of income needed, and the need to deal with business aspects. Various resources provide guidance for freelance editors.
- Both medicine and editing are continually changing fields. Various resources can aid in keeping up.
- Satisfactions of a medical editing career include continual learning; interaction with bright, interesting people; the joys of solving puzzles and helping to create well-crafted products; and, perhaps especially, the chance to serve authors, publishers, readers, and ultimately patients through this helping profession.

Acknowledgments

As fellow editors know, even a single-authored book reflects the contributions of many people. I am grateful to all who contributed directly or indirectly to this book.

Special thanks go to Mary Laur, acquisitions editor for the Chicago Guides to Writing, Editing, and Publishing series; to the peer reviewers of the proposal and manuscript for this book; and to Madison V. Brown and Laura Larocca, who reviewed the manuscript from an early-career standpoint. Also deeply appreciated are the contributions of others at or engaged by the University of Chicago Press, including senior editorial associate Andrea Blatz, production editor Elizabeth Ellingboe, manuscript editor Marianne Tatom, and designer Daniel Goldberg. I am thankful as well to indexer Tobiah Waldron and promotions and marketing communications director Carrie Olivia Adams.

I also am grateful to the students whose questions, misinterpretations, or puzzled looks led me to develop or refine explanations that now appear in this book. I am grateful as well to colleagues—including those in the American Medical Writers Association, the Council of Science Editors, and other professional groups—from whom I have learned much. Likewise, I am indebted to the administrators who have supported me in a career embodying my affinities for both medical content and the editor's craft.

As I hope this book shows, the medical editor's craft draws on much more than medical acquaintance and language-related skills. Therefore, I am grateful to those, including my parents and various teachers, who have encouraged me to always keep learning, to think critically, to solve problems creatively, to maintain the highest ethical standards, and to treat others with respect and kindness. Such attributes, I believe, help distinguish the exemplary editor.

Finally, I thank my husband, Thomas I. Vogel, for everything over the years. To him I dedicate this book.

· APPENDIX 1 ·

Creating and Using a Style Sheet for an Abstract

Below is a fictional example of an abstract of the type that could accompany a journal article or conference presentation. It is followed by an example of a style sheet that might be created from editing it and then by a copy of the abstract as it could be edited in keeping with the style sheet.

Unedited Fictional Abstract

Treatment of Editors' Disease; A Randomized Trial

Background. Editors' disease effects approximately 2/3 of professional manuscript editor's. Common manifestations include: cephalgia, xeropthalmia, kyphosis, hyperphagia or anorexia and anxiety. Small studies that have been done previously suggest that Valium, cream sherry, yoga, and dark choclate each may alleviate editors' disease.

Methods. 1000 American Medical Writers' Association members who were medical editors with editors' disease were randomly assigned to receive 5 mg of diazepam twice every day, 100 milliliters of Cream Sherry every evening, a yoga class 3 times per week, one ounce per day of 85 percent cocoa dark chocolate or no intervention. Before the trial and then again after 12 weeks, a team of two nurses determined an EDIT (Editors' Disease International Test) score for each and every participant. In addition to this, editorial productivity also was monitered during the study that we undertook.

Results. 912 of the editers completed the trial. Completion rates did not exhibit any significant differences among groups (*P*=0.92). All 6 groups, including the control group, showed some improvement in EDIT score over the 12 weeks. In the dark-chocolate group, all but three members (who reported substituting Sneakers bars for dark chocolate) showed full recovery (final EDIT test score of 0). Rates of full recovery in the other groups ranged from 21-23%. The differences in recovery rate between the dark-chocolate group and the other groups were highly significant (*P* >237%). We think this finding was because editors love chocolate. The Diazepam and cream sherry groups showed slightly lower productivity then the other groups.

Conclusions. Dark chocolate cured editor's disease in this group of medical editors that we studied. It's effectiveness should undergo assessment in other editorial populations.

Style Sheet for Fictional Abstract

AUTHOR/TITLE	Izzy Investigator et al./ Treatment of Editors' Disease: A Randomized Trial
COPYEDITOR	Elliott Editor
DATE	February 14, 2025
REFERENCES	*AMA Manual of Style*, 11th edition *Merriam-Webster's Collegiate Dictionary*, 11th ed. (https://merriam-webster.com) Instructions to authors: *Pretend Medical Journal* (https://pmedj.org/instr)

PUNCTUATION

- Use serial comma (example: a, b, and c).
- No colon between a verb (such as *include*) and a list that follows.

NUMBER STYLE

- Generally use numerals even for numbers less than 10 (example: 5 groups).
- Do not begin a sentence with a numeral.

- Hyphenate common fractions (example: two-thirds).
- Use the % sign, not the word *percent*.
- For percentage ranges, connect the percentages with *to* and place the % sign after each number (example: 21% to 23%).
- Place a space before and a space after operators such as plus signs and equal signs.
- *P* values should not have a zero before the decimal point.

OTHER

- Use generic rather than brand names. Do not capitalize generic names.
- Use metric units. Abbreviate names of units when they follow numbers.
- If an acronym will be used, write out the term in full, followed by the acronym in parentheses, on first appearance.

ALPHABETICAL LIST OF TERMS

American Medical Writers Association (without an apostrophe)
anorexia
cephalgia
diazepam
editors' disease (with an apostrophe at the end)
Editors' Disease International Test (EDIT)
hyperphagia
kyphosis
P (to indicate *P* value)
Snickers bars
xerophthalmia
yoga

Edited Version of Fictional Abstract

In the version below, mechanical errors have been corrected, discrepancies with the style sheet have been resolved, the wording has been made more concise, and the author has been queried where warranted.

Treatment of Editors' Disease~~;~~: A Randomized Trial

Background. Editors' disease ~~effects~~affects approximately ~~2/3~~two-thirds of professional manuscript editor~~'~~s. Common manifestations include~~:~~ cephalgia, xerophthalmia, kyphosis, hyperphagia or anorexia, and anxiety. Small studies ~~that have been done previously~~ suggest that ~~Valium~~diazepam, cream sherry, yoga, and dark chocolate each may alleviate editors' disease.

Methods. ~~1000~~One thousand American Medical Writers' Association members who were medical editors with editors' disease were randomly assigned to receive 5 mg of diazepam twice ~~every day~~daily, 100 ~~milliliters~~ml of ~~Cream Sherry~~cream sherry every evening, a yoga class 3 times per week, one ounce per day of 85 percent cocoa dark chocolate, or no intervention. Before the trial and ~~then again~~ after 12 weeks, a team of ~~two~~2 nurses determined an ~~EDIT (~~Editors' Disease International Test~~)~~ (EDIT) score for each ~~and every~~ participant. ~~In addition to this, e~~Editorial productivity also was ~~moniterered~~monitored. ~~during the study that we undertook.~~

Results. Of the editors, 912 ~~of the editors~~ completed the trial. Completion rates did not ~~exhibit any significant differences~~differ significantly among groups ($P = 0.92$). All 6 groups, including the control group, showed some improvement in EDIT score over the 12 weeks. In the dark-chocolate group, all but ~~three~~3 members (who reported substituting ~~Sneakers~~Snickers bars for dark chocolate) showed full recovery (final EDIT ~~test~~ score of 0). Rates of full recovery in the other groups ranged from ~~21–23%~~21% to 23%. The differences in recovery rate between the dark-chocolate group and the other groups were highly significant ($P > 237\%$). We think this finding was because editors love chocolate. The ~~Diazepam~~diazepam and cream sherry groups showed slightly lower productivity ~~then~~than the other groups.

Conclusions. Dark chocolate cured ~~editor's~~editors' disease in this group of medical editors ~~that we studied~~. ~~It's~~Its effectiveness should ~~undergo assessment~~be assessed in other editorial populations.

Commented [Editor]: Thank you for having me edit your abstract, which I found informative and generally well organized. My edits appear in Track Changes in the text, and my queries are in comment bubbles below. If you have questions, please feel free to ask.

Commented [Editor]: Please check whether this comma placement retains the intended meaning.

Commented [Editor]: Usual practice in such abstracts is to use metric units. Perhaps convert ounces to grams.

Commented [Editor]: Above, 5 groups are noted. Please resolve the discrepancy.

Commented [Editor]: Please check: Was Snickers (not Sneakers) meant?

Commented [Editor]: Please check, as P values are not percentages and cannot exceed 1.

Commented [Editor]: This statement is a comment, not a finding. Therefore, if it is retained, it should be moved to the Conclusions section.

Commented [Editor]: Might "cured" be too strong a term?(It seems unclear whether the dark chocolate cured the condition permanently.) Perhaps use wording such as "fully alleviated."

· APPENDIX 2 ·

A Style Sheet for an Article for General Readers

AUTHOR/WORKING TITLE	Barbara Gastel/Fauci: Who and Why
COPYEDITOR	Evelyn Editter
DATE	March 15, 2025
REFERENCES	AP Stylebook, Merriam-Webster dictionary

PUNCTUATION

No serial comma (example: a, b and c)
TV program names in quotation marks (example: "Saturday Night Live")
Space on each side of dash

NUMBER STYLE

In general, spell out one through nine.
Figures for 1 through 9 for ages and before units of measure
Dates (example: Dec. 24, 1940)
1980s
Ordinal numbers: no superscript (example: 32nd)

Based on "10 reasons why Anthony Fauci was ready to be the face of the US pandemic response" (https://theconversation.com/10-reasons-why-anthony-fauci-was-ready-to-be-the-face-of-the-us-pandemic-response-150596).

OTHER

- "Dr." before first reference to a given physician. On subsequent mentions, only surname.
- Don't put the acronym (example: NIH) in parentheses after the first use of the full term.
- Don't italicize names of magazines and journals (example: Time magazine).

ALPHABETICAL LIST OF NAMES/TERMS

AIDS (OK to use without spelling out first)
Anthony S. Fauci
Brad Pitt
College of the Holy Cross
COVID-19
Ebola
granulomatosis
Larry Kramer
National Institute of Allergy and Infectious Diseases
National Institutes of Health
New England Journal of Medicine
NIH
PEPFAR
polyangiitis
President George W. Bush
President's Emergency Plan for AIDS Relief
Proceedings of the National Academy of Sciences
Regis High
SARS
Saturday Night Live
T-shirt
U.S.
U.S. Public Health Service
Vietnam
Washington Post
Zika

Answer Keys: Exercises

Some Sentences to Copyedit

This key shows suitable copyediting of the sentences in this exercise. In some places, slightly different edits also may be acceptable.

Please copyedit the following sentences. Do not make any other changes. AMA style should be followed insofar as feasible.

1. Of the 47 ~~diabetics~~people with diabetes ~~confined to~~who used wheelchairs, 23 (~~48.9361~~49%) ~~utilized~~used ~~I~~ibuprofen.
2. According to ~~HIPPA~~HIPAA, ~~PA's~~PAs should not reveal such information about the ~~cases~~patients they treat.
3. This ~~67-year old~~67-year-old ~~female~~woman with Parkinson~~'s~~ ~~D~~disease also ~~suffered from~~had ~~I~~irritable ~~B~~bowel ~~S~~syndrome (IBS), which ~~lead~~led her to consult our clinic.
4. Signs and ~~S~~symptoms of this disease include~~:~~ fever, fatigue, and a distinctive rash.
5. This year, 4 students will report on ~~Staphylococcus Aureus~~*Staphylococcus aureus* during the unit on ~~preventative~~preventive medicine.
6. In total, 274 ~~b~~Black patients met all the inclusion ~~criterion~~criteria for the study.

7. Her main mentor, Dr. Li, helped her design the research, and her ~~writing-instructor~~writing instructor helped her edit the resulting paper.
8. While he was ~~W~~waiting for the bus, his foot began to ache, his skin began to itch, and ~~twitching of~~ his ears ~~started~~began to twitch.
9. The day before the procedure~~;~~, you should ~~only~~ consume only clear liquids such as lemon-lime ~~gateraid~~Gatorade.
10. Because this test often fails to detect cases, researchers at the National Institutes of Health ~~[NEH]~~(NIH) are trying to ~~device~~devise one with greater ~~specificity~~sensitivity.

Organization of a Journal Article

This key indicates the journal article section in which each statement appears most likely to occur. In some contexts, some of the sentences also might appear in other sections.

Substantive editors of journal articles reporting medical research must assess whether statements are in the correct section. Please write I, M, R, or D after each sentence to indicate whether it is likely to fit best in the introduction, methods section, results section, or discussion.

1. The objective of our study was to determine whether Procedure A is superior to Procedure B. **I**
2. Whole-genome sequencing was performed with the use of Illumina MiSeq. **M**
3. All deaths were classified by using the International Classification of Diseases, 11th Revision. **M**
4. Future studies should quantify the magnitude of this type of activity. **D**
5. Of the 3478 screening swabs, 183 (5.3%) yielded one or more isolates. **R**
6. ______ is an emerging pathogen that has recently been associated with outbreaks worldwide. **I**
7. Participants aged 25 to 50 years who were referred to 1 of 6 participating hospitals were eligible for inclusion. **M**
8. Our findings are consistent with the pooled results of earlier trials. **D**
9. In total, 120 (40%) of the 300 nurses responded to questions in the survey. **R**

10. Our current study has several limitations. **D**
11. RNA was isolated by Hinton method II (39). **M**
12. Our results indicate that reusable patient equipment may serve as a source of health care-associated outbreaks of infection with this agent. **D**
13. We emailed the survey to 375 academic authors in September 2024. **M**
14. Figure 3 shows the changes in function during the 2-year follow-up period. **R**
15. The findings of our current study add to the body of research showing an association between ____ and ____. **D**
16. Twelve dogs in the XYZ group and 11 dogs in the control group had complete healing at the 2-week reevaluation. **R**
17. The Student *t* test was used to identify differences between groups. **M**
18. The healing rate resembled that in a previous study of this intervention. **D**
19. Significantly lower rates were found in patients with ABC ($P = .024$). **R**
20. Our hypothesis was that ___ may predispose patients with XYZ to develop cancer. **I**
21. This finding is in complete contrast to our expectation. **D**
22. Patients were stratified by sex and by ethnic group. **M**
23. Another possible explanation for this finding may be related to continuous treatment with ______. **D**
24. After autoradiography, films were scanned using a Powerlook 100XL densitometer (Bio-Rad). **M**
25. These findings are especially interesting in the context of HIV vaccine development. **D**

Providing Substantive Feedback on an Abstract

This key indicates strengths of the fictional draft abstract and suggestions for improvement. Slightly different lists of strengths and suggestions also may be acceptable.

SOME CURRENT STRENGTHS OF THE DRAFT

The draft has a suitable overall structure. In general, it is clear and concise. It also seems to be a suitable length.

SOME SUGGESTIONS

(These suggestions are listed by sentence number.)

2. Because abstracts often appear without the paper they summarize, they should not cite references.
3. For clarity, and in keeping with current norms, "the authors" should be "we."
3. For conciseness, perhaps reword "undertook a study of ways to improve abstracts accompanying papers that are submitted to medical journals" as "studied ways to improve papers submitted to medical journals."
4. It would be helpful to provide more information about the methods—for example, how many researchers were studied, how many medical centers they came from, and whether they were randomly assigned to the various groups.
5. Please indicate what GOKW stands for. If not clear from the name, perhaps briefly note the nature of this rubric. [Note from author of exercise: Here, GOKW stands for "God Only Knows What."]
6. If it is to be stated here that the journal editors were asked to rate the abstract, the results section of the abstract should indicate the main finding(s) in this regard.
7. These statistical procedures are so common that they need not be mentioned in an abstract.
8. The phrase "when compared to" can be condensed to "than."
8. Because abstracts often appear without the paper they summarize, tables should not be cited.
8. It would be helpful to say how much higher this group scored and to provide an indicator of statistical significance (for example, a *P* value).
10. If interview results are to be noted here, the methods section should indicate that interviews were done.
11. Because this content is commentary, it should go in the conclusions section if it is retained.
12. This sentence seems tangential. The conclusions section should focus on presenting conclusions, drawn from the current research, regarding the main subject of the study (in this case, ways to improve abstracts).
13. This sentence presents a finding. Therefore, if it is retained, it belongs in the results section.

15. Although it is important to be transparent about funding sources, such sources normally are not mentioned in abstracts.

Editing for Conciseness

This key shows suitable editing of the sentences for conciseness. Care was taken not to change the meaning. In some places, slightly different edits also may be acceptable.

Condense the wordy part of each of the following sentences. Do not make other changes. Take care not to change meaning.

1. ~~The majority of~~Most nurses report this problem.
2. They completed the task ~~in an efficient manner~~efficiently.
3. Editing ~~has the potential to~~can improve text.
4. The procedure ~~produced an increase in~~increased the rate.
5. ~~Despite the fact that~~Although he took the course, he edits poorly.
   or Despite ~~the fact that he took~~taking the course, he edits poorly.
6. Next we counted the ~~number of~~ cells.
7. Patients of many ~~different~~ nationalities attend the clinic.
8. The lesion was green ~~in color~~.
9. She discussed advances in ~~the field of~~ neurology.
10. They should exercise ~~on a~~ daily ~~basis~~.

Some Cases to Consider

The 10 ethics cases at the end of chapter 8 are briefly discussed below. The discussions are not answer keys per se, because considerations can differ depending on circumstances and because more than one reasonable approach can exist. However, the discussions demonstrate types of aspects and approaches to consider. Recurrent themes include asking for clarifications rather than jumping to accusations, communicating tactfully, using situations as chances to educate, and suggesting constructive alternatives to questionable actions.

CASE 1: SUSPICIOUSLY SAME?

You are editing a grant proposal by a non-native user of English. In general, the prose is clear but not entirely idiomatic. However, you encounter a paragraph in which the prose is very polished. On pasting the paragraph into Google, you find that it is the same as in a published paper that the author cites. What do you think is happening here? How do you approach the situation? Why?

Discussion: The duplication might have occurred for any of several reasons. For example, maybe the author meant to paraphrase but forgot to do so, maybe the author comes from a culture where such duplication is acceptable, or maybe the author is struggling with the language. Rather than speculating or accusing, it can be advisable to point out the duplication to the author and nonconfrontationally ask how it occurred. Depending on the response, you might then, for instance, clarify norms and offer to help with paraphrasing. In the unlikely event that the author insists on retaining the paragraph as is, consider indicating that you will inform their supervisor.

CASE 2: CONCEALED CONFLICTS?

You are editing a paper about a new medical device. The section where the authors should identify conflicts of interest states that none of the authors have conflicts of interest regarding the current research. However, you know that two of the authors are consultants to the company that manufactures the device. What do you think is happening here? How do you proceed? Why?

Discussion: This situation might have occurred for various reasons. Perhaps the authors believe they do not have a conflict of interest because they do not think the consulting influenced their judgment. Or perhaps the authors worry that reporting a conflict of interest will decrease the likelihood that the paper will be considered or published. Or maybe your recollection is incorrect. Quite likely, the best approach in this instance is to nonconfrontationally share your perception that a conflict of interest may exist. If the reply then warrants, clarification can follow regarding the definition of conflict of interest and the fact that declaring such conflicts does not preclude review and publication.

CASE 3: DÉJÀ VU?

As a manuscript editor at a medical journal, you find that an image provided as evidence in the results section of a manuscript seems strangely familiar. Upon checking, you see that it appeared in the results section of the author's previously published paper in your journal—allegedly about a different experiment. What do you think might have happened? How do you proceed? Why?

Discussion: This duplication might have occurred in either of two main ways. Perhaps the author carelessly submitted the incorrect image. More seriously, perhaps the author fabricated the findings and used an existing image to support them. Because a serious ethical infraction might have occurred, it probably would be best to report your observation to your supervisor (such as the head of the manuscript editing group or the editor-in-chief), who can then decide how to proceed.

CASE 4: TOO FAST?

As an author's editor, you are reviewing a peer reviewer's report with an author and discussing how to proceed. The reviewer has said the author should do an additional experiment and add the results to the paper. However, the author protests that doing so would be too much work. Two hours later, the author returns with a version of the paper that includes the results of the requested experiment. What do you think has happened? How do you proceed? Why?

Discussion: The speed with which the results were produced and reported suggests that they were fabricated. It therefore seems advisable to ask the author how the results were obtained so fast. If it seems that the results were indeed fabricated, an author's editor should try to persuade the author not to submit them; if the author insists on doing so, informing the author's supervisor is likely to be in order. Also, the author might not know that reviewers' requests can be challenged if sound scientific reasons exist for doing so. As an author's editor, you may be of service by noting this fact and offering to help the author craft a respectful, persuasive rebuttal.

CASE 5: ABOVE AND BEYOND?

The findings of a major clinical study are about to be published in a journal. As an editor at the institution where the study was done, you are editing a news release about the findings. It appears to you that the draft of the release overstates one of the main findings of the study. Why might the seeming overstatement have occurred? How do you proceed? Why?

Discussion: The seeming overstatement might reflect any of three main factors. Perhaps the person writing the release misunderstood the research. (Often, people writing news releases have little science background.) Perhaps the person writing the release mistakenly believed that exaggerating the findings would help promote the institution. Or perhaps you yourself incorrectly perceived that there was an overstatement. A first step would be to review the findings again to see whether an overstatement indeed seems to have occurred. If there does seem to be an overstatement, you should correct it (ideally in collaboration with the writer) before the release goes out. If it is unclear from the materials available whether the finding was overstated, consulting a main author of the journal article would be advisable.

CASE 6: OVERLY APPRECIATIVE?

You are a member of the editorial office at a medical research institute. A large grant proposal that you edited has been accepted, and the principal investigator (PI) is thrilled. On opening a thank-you note that the PI sends you, you find that it contains a very large gift certificate to a luxury clothing store. How do you react? How do you proceed? Why?

Discussion: Some institutions or offices have a policy on accepting gifts. If yours does, consult it and proceed accordingly, which typically would entail declining the large gift. In doing so, you could cite the policy but say you were glad the PI appreciated your work. If no policy exists, returning a large gift still is highly advisable, in part because such a gift may carry expectations of favors—editorial or otherwise. In tactfully declining the gift, you can note that professional norms call for doing so. In some circumstances, you may be able to suggest that the sum be donated to charity or, for example, to your office's professional-development fund.

CASE 7: WHOSE VIEWS?

You are a postdoctoral fellow hoping to pursue a medical editing career. The scientist heading the laboratory in which you work has agreed to peer-review a journal article but is very busy. Knowing your interests, the scientist asks you to do the peer review and submit it on their behalf. What do you think of the idea? How do you proceed? Why?

Discussion: Gaining experience in peer reviewing can aid a prospective editor. However, manuscripts for peer review are confidential and so should not be shared. Also, submitting a review under someone else's name is dishonest. The best approach probably would be to ask that the scientist request the journal's permission for you to do the review (or, perhaps better, to request the journal's permission for you to collaborate on the review, so you can learn more from the experience and the journal can benefit from some input from the scientist). Quite likely, the journal will grant permission. However, proceeding without the permission would not be ethical.

CASE 8: FREE ADVICE?

You are an author's editor at a health science center, and an ambitious graduate student approaches you with an idea. First, they say, they will submit the paper to the regional biomedical journal. Then, after receiving the peer reviews, they will withdraw the paper, use the peer reviews to improve it, and submit the paper to a higher-ranking journal. What do you think of the idea? How do you proceed? Why?

Discussion: The graduate student's idea is dreadful. Submitting a paper to a journal entails committing to publishing it there if accepted. The student's proposed behavior would waste the time of editors and reviewers and would violate trust. This behavior also could mar the student's reputation with journals, and it could backfire if the higher-ranking journal chose a peer reviewer who had reviewed the paper for the regional journal. A good approach might be to compliment the student on their commitment to obtaining feedback and to propose acceptable ways of doing so. Such ways include requesting pre-submission feedback from other researchers and, of course, using the author's editing service available at the health science center.

CASE 9: EXTRA EDITING?

You are a freelance medical editor doing some author's editing for an editing company. A manuscript seems excellent overall, and so you make few editorial changes. On receiving the edited manuscript, your contact at the editing company says you should make more changes so the authors feel they are getting their money's worth. What do you think? How do you proceed?

Discussion: Good editing does not necessarily entail making many editorial changes, just as a good medical examination need not result in prescribing many drugs. Editorial changes should not be made just to show that the manuscript was thoroughly reviewed. Indeed, arbitrary changes can harm a manuscript and undermine authors' confidence in the editing. Ideally, these points should be made to the contact at the editing company. If evidence that the editorial review has been thorough is sought, you may be able to list aspects that you reviewed, provide a copy of the edited manuscript containing some comments on items done well, or both. Ultimately, if the editing company persists in equating thoroughness of editing with number of changes made, it might be best to avoid working for that company.

CASE 10: EXTRA CREDIT?

You have edited a manuscript to submit to a journal. Your editing has consisted mainly of correcting mechanical errors, increasing consistency with the journal's style, improving some of the organization, making some reasoning clearer, ensuring that references are cited where needed, and streamlining the language. The lead author is delighted with your work and offers to list you as an author. What do you think of the idea? What do you say to the lead author? Why?

Discussion: From the description, you have copyedited and substantively edited the manuscript. You therefore deserve acknowledgment. However, your contributions are not of types that qualify for authorship. Also, authorship entails taking ethical responsibility for the research—a responsibility you might not be ready to accept. Therefore, the best approach is to express appreciation of the offer, note that your contributions do not meet the criteria for authorship, and ask that you be listed in the acknowledgments instead; you could offer to propose wording for this acknowledgment. If you work in an editorial office, you also could say you would be pleased to have the lead author commend you to your supervisor. In addition, you might keep the lead editor in mind as a potential reference, in case later you apply for a new job or are nominated for an award. Likewise, if you are a freelance editor, you could encourage the lead author to provide additional work, recommend you to others, and perhaps provide a testimonial for your website. And maybe on days when your editing seems unappreciated, you can think back on how delighted this author was with your work.

Abbreviations

AADEJ · American Association of Dental Editors and Journalists
ACES · ACES: The Society for Editing
ACS · American Chemical Society
AHCJ · Association of Health Care Journalists
AI · artificial intelligence
AMA · American Medical Association
AMWA · American Medical Writers Association
AP · Associated Press
APA · American Psychological Association
ARRIVE · Animal Research: Reporting of In Vivo Experiments
BELS · Board of Editors in the Life Sciences
CARE · CAse REports
CDC · Centers for Disease Control and Prevention
CME · continuing medical education
CMPP · Certified Medical Publication Professional
CONSORT · Consolidated Standards of Reporting Trials
COPE · Committee on Publication Ethics
CRediT · Contributor Role Taxonomy
CSE · Council of Science Editors
CV · curriculum vitae
DIA · Drug Information Association
EASE · European Association of Science Editors

EFA · Editorial Freelancers Association
EQUATOR Network · Enhancing the QUAlity and Transparency Of health Research Network
HIPAA · Health Insurance Portability and Accountability Act
IACUC · institutional animal care and use committee
ICMJE · International Committee of Medical Journal Editors
IMRAD format · introduction, methods, results, and discussion
INANE · International Academy of Nursing Editors
IRB · institutional review board
ISMPP · International Society for Medical Publication Professionals
IT · information technology
JAMA · *Journal of the American Medical Association*
MOOC · massive open online course
MWC · Medical Writer Certified
NASW · National Association of Science Writers
NIH · National Institutes of Health
OWL · Purdue University Online Writing Lab
PDF · portable document format
PI · principal investigator
PRISMA · Preferred Reporting Items for Systematic reviews and Meta-Analyses
QR CODE · quick response code
RAPS · Regulatory Affairs Professionals Society
ScENe · Scientific Editors Network
SRQR · Standards for Reporting Qualitative Research
STROBE · STrengthening the Reporting of OBservational studies in Epidemiology
URL · uniform resource locator
WAME · World Association of Medical Editors

Glossary

abbreviation. Shortened form of a word or phrase. Used in place of the full word or phrase.

acquisitions editor. An editor in charge of acquiring manuscripts for a book publisher.

acronym. Abbreviation formed from the first letters of some or all words in a phrase.

alt text. Short for *alternative text*. Text, usually hidden from regular view, that describes an image for users such as people with visual disabilities who use screen readers.

author's editor. An editor working directly with authors to refine their writing before submission.

billboard paragraph. See **nut graf**.

biosketch. Short for *biographical sketch*. In the broad sense, a brief piece of writing that summarizes a person's experience and qualifications. In the narrow sense, a document providing, in a required format, biographical information on a person seeking a grant or listed in a grant application as part of the proposed project team.

caption. The text accompanying an illustration or a photograph.

case report. A journal article describing and discussing a noteworthy clinical case.

certificate. Documentation that a person has successfully completed a given set of educational activities.

certification. Documentation that a person has demonstrated proficiency, for example by passing a standardized examination.

conflict of interest. A situation in which a concurrent involvement has the potential to bias an individual's judgment.

contributor. Someone who participated in producing the research reported in a scientific paper or in the writing of the paper. May or may not qualify for listing as an author.

copyediting. In the broad sense, *copyediting* is a synonym for *manuscript editing*. In its narrow sense, copyediting is refining written material to ensure proper mechanics (such as grammar, spelling, and word usage) and compliance with the publisher's style (such as conventions being followed for punctuation, number format, and reference format); it also can include improving the formatting of figures and tables.

copyeditor. An editor who refines written materials. Also known as a **manuscript editor**.

corresponding author. For papers with more than one author, the author who communicates with the journal to which the paper is submitted.

curriculum vitae. (Plural: *curricula vitae*.) The academic counterpart to a resume. Tends to be considerably longer than a resume and, for example, to list all journal articles by the individual.

deck. Blurb under the title of a journalistic article.

desk reject. Informal term for a journal's rejection of a paper without having it undergo peer review.

DOI. Digital object identifier. An identification code, assigned to an online item, that provides a persistent link to its location on the internet.

editor-in-chief. The editor in charge of a publication.

fabrication. Making up (inventing) findings rather than obtaining them through scientific research. A major ethical violation.

fact-checking. Checking a document to ensure that every piece of information in it is correct and that the overall message is accurate.

falsification. Changing findings or omitting relevant ones, thus resulting in inaccurate reporting of research. A major ethical violation.

feature article. A journalistic article that, rather than reporting news, focuses on a topic or person. Also known as a *feature story*.

ghost author. An individual whose contributions merit listing as an author but who is not listed.

grant proposal. A proposal describing work for which funding is being sought. Also known as a *grant application*.

graphical abstract. See **visual abstract.**

guest author. An individual who is listed as an author but who has not contributed sufficiently to the work to merit listing.

IMRAD structure. The typical structure of a scientific paper. Stands for **I**ntroduction, **M**ethods, **R**esults, **a**nd **D**iscussion.

institutional animal care and use committee. Committee that reviews proposed research on animals to ensure that it complies with ethical standards. Commonly referred to as an IACUC.

institutional review board. Committee that reviews proposed research on human subjects to ensure that it complies with ethical standards. Commonly referred to as an IRB.

instructions to authors. A set of instructions regarding the content and format of papers to be submitted to a given journal. Appears on the journal's website.

inverted pyramid format. Typical format for a news story in the popular press. Begins with the main point; progressively finer details follow.

keywords. Terms identifying the main topics of an article.

legend. The text accompanying a figure or other visual.

level of editing. Intensity with which a document is edited. For example, light editing focuses largely on mechanics (such as grammar, spelling, and punctuation); medium editing addresses items such as conciseness as well; and heavy editing also regards items such as organization. Note that the level of editing designates only the types of changes made, not the number of changes made.

macroediting. Editing focusing mainly on overall content and organization.

managing editor. An editor responsible for administrative aspects of a publication.

manuscript. The unpublished form of a paper or other piece of writing.

manuscript editor. An editor who refines written materials. Also known as a **copyeditor.**

microediting. Editing for detail, largely at the sentence level.

multi-language author. Author who uses more than one language. Often used to refer to authors writing in English as a foreign language.

news release. A news article prepared by an institution and disseminated to members of the popular media, either to publish as is or to generate coverage. Also known as a **press release.**

nut graf. Short for *nutshell paragraph*. A paragraph, early in a feature article, that indicates the focus and scope of the article. Also called a **billboard paragraph.**

orphan. Single line of type at the bottom of a column. Considered undesirable in page design.

parallelism. Use of the same grammatical form for all items in a series.

peer review. The process of having subject-matter experts evaluate submissions. Items commonly undergoing peer review include journal submissions and grant proposals.

peer reviewer. A subject-matter specialist providing peer review. Sometimes also known as a **referee.**

personal statement. An application essay, commonly indicating the applicant's background, interests, and goals. Also sometimes called a **statement of purpose.**

pitch. See **query letter.**

plagiarism. Presenting others' words or ideas as one's own rather than crediting the source. A major ethical violation.

point of entry. Element in a journalistic article that initially attracts those browsing to read it.

preprint. A paper that is posted online before, or instead of, being submitted to a journal.

preprint server. A website devoted to hosting preprints.

press release. See **news release.**

principal investigator. A researcher taking the lead on a project (or set of projects) and obtaining the funding to conduct it. Often referred to as a PI (pronounced "pee-eye").

proceedings. A document consisting mainly of papers presented at a conference.

production editor. An editor coordinating the process of transforming an accepted manuscript into a published piece.

proof. A copy of material as it is to look when it is published. Authors receive a proof to check for problems such as typographical errors.

proofreading. Final checking of written material for typographical and other errors.

public information officer. A communication specialist employed by an institution (such as a university or government agency) to disseminate information to the public.

pull quotes. Article excerpts that are set in larger type to serve as a design element and to draw readers in.

QR code. Short for quick response code. A two-dimensional barcode, typically used to link to a website.

query. A written question from a manuscript editor to an author, for example about an inconsistency, ambiguity, or missing item.

query letter. A letter or message, generally from a freelance writer, proposing an article to an outlet such as a magazine. Also known as a **pitch.**

referee. See **peer reviewer.**

review article. An article summarizing and integrating the literature on a given topic.

running title. A shortened version of an article title, commonly appearing at the tops of pages.

salami science. Dividing between two or more papers the research findings that should appear in a single paper.

science writing. Writing that is about science and intended for general readers.

scientific editor. An editor responsible for scientific content of a publication. At medical journals, scientific editors typically are active medical researchers rather than professional editors.

scientific paper. An article, typically published in a journal, reporting new research. Usually consists mainly of an introduction, a methods section, a results section, and a discussion.

scientific writing. Writing about science that is by scientists and intended for fellow scientists. Examples include scientific papers and grant proposals.

sidebar. Short related article accompanying and complementing the main article.

stacked nouns. A series of consecutive nouns without intervening prepositions, such that the relationship among the nouns is unclear.

statement of purpose. See **personal statement.**

structured abstract. An abstract containing standardized headings, generally corresponding to respective parts of a scientific paper.

study section. A committee peer-reviewing grant proposals submitted to the (US) National Institutes of Health.

style. Set of conventions followed by a given publication, for example regarding punctuation, capitalization, and number format. An example is AMA (American Medical Association) style, presented in the *AMA Manual of Style.*

style manual. Book providing copyeditorial and other guidelines to follow in writing and editing. Can be general or geared to conventions in a specific field or genre.

substantive editing. Refining written material to improve content and organization.

summary lead. Typical beginning of a news story, consisting of a brief statement of the story's main message.

syntax. The way in which words, phrases, or other such elements of language are arranged.

tagging. Inserting codes in a document to delineate types of elements, such as headings, in order to guide design.

text recycling. Including the same text in more than one publication.

visual abstract. A visual summary of a paper, commonly focusing largely on key findings. Also called a **graphical abstract**.

widow. Single line of type at the top of a column. Considered undesirable in page design.

References

AMA Manual of Style Committee. 2020. *AMA Manual of Style: A Guide for Authors and Editors*. 11th ed. Oxford University Press.

American Medical Writers Association. n.d. "AMWA Code of Ethics." https://cdn.ymaws.com/www.amwa.org/resource/resmgr/membership/amwa_code_of_ethics.pdf.

American Psychological Association. 2020. *Publication Manual of the American Psychological Association*. 7th ed. American Psychological Association.

Annesley, Thomas M. 2010a. "Put Your Best Figure Forward: Line Graphs and Scattergrams." *Clinical Chemistry* 56 (8): 1229–33. https://doi.org/10.1373/clinchem.2010.150060.

Annesley, Thomas M. 2010b. "Bars and Pies Make Better Desserts Than Figures." *Clinical Chemistry* 56 (9): 1394–1400. https://doi.org/10.1373/clinchem.2010.152298.

Annesley, Thomas M. 2010c. "Bring Your Best to the Table." *Clinical Chemistry* 56 (10): 1528–34. https://doi.org/10.1373/clinchem.2010.153502.

[Annesley, Thomas M., and Pamela A. Derish.] [2010–2011.] Clinical Chemistry *Guide to Scientific Writing*. https://academic.oup.com/clinchem/pages/guide-to-scientific-writing.

Associated Press. 2024. *The Associated Press Stylebook*. 57th ed. Associated Press.

Banik, Gregory M., Grace Baysinger, Prashant V. Kamat, and Norbert J. Pienta, eds. 2020. *ACS Guide to Scholarly Communication*. American Chemical Society. https://pubs.acs.org/doi/book/10.1021/acsguide.

Berg, A. Scott. 1978. *Max Perkins: Editor of Genius*. Dutton.

Bird, Stephanie J., Mohammad Hosseini, and Dena K. Plemmons. 2023. *Authors*

Without Borders: Guidelines for Discussing Authorship with Collaborators. Sigma Xi, the Scientific Honor Society. https://online.fliphtml5.com/oaiev/cipo/.

Board of Editors in the Life Sciences. 2024. "Board of Editors in the Life Sciences Code of Ethics." https://bels.memberclicks.net/code-of-ethics2.

Boettger, Ryan K. 2012. "Types of Errors Used in Medical Editing Tests." *AMWA Journal* 27 (3): 99–104.

Borel, Brooke. 2023. *The Chicago Guide to Fact-Checking*. 2nd ed. University of Chicago Press.

Brenner, Erin. 2024. *The Chicago Guide for Freelance Editors: How to Take Care of Your Business, Your Clients, and Yourself from Start-Up to Sustainability*. University of Chicago Press.

Bűky, Erika, Marilyn Schwartz, and Amy Einsohn. 2019. *The Copyeditor's Workbook: Exercises and Tips for Honing Your Editorial Judgment*. University of California Press.

Churchill, R. Elliott. 2001. "Microediting." In *Essays for Biomedical Communicators: Volume 1 of Selected AMWA Workshops*, edited by Florence M. Witte and Nancy Dew Taylor, 117–26. American Medical Writers Association.

Churchill, R. Elliott, Martha M. Tacker, and Frances H. Porcher. 2001. "Macroediting." In *Essays for Biomedical Communicators: Volume 1 of Selected AMWA Workshops*, edited by Florence M. Witte and Nancy Dew Taylor, 127–32. American Medical Writers Association.

Committee on Science, Engineering, and Public Policy, National Academy of Science, National Academy of Engineering, and Institute of Medicine of the National Academies. 2009. *On Being a Scientist: A Guide to Responsible Conduct in Research*. 3rd ed. National Academies Press. https://nap.nationalacademies.org/catalog/12192/on-being-a-scientist-a-guide-to-responsible-conduct-in.

Conners, Deanna Erin. 2024. *Avoiding Common Pitfalls in Medical Writing: An Editor's Advice*. Milne Open Textbooks. https://milneopentextbooks.org/avoiding-common-pitfalls-in-medical-writing/.

Council of Science Editors Editorial Policy Committee. n.d. *Recommendations for Promoting Integrity in Scientific Journal Publications*. https://www.councilscienceeditors.org/recommendations-for-promoting-integrity-in-scientific-journal-publications.

Council of Science Editors Style Manual Task Force. 2024. *The CSE Manual: Scientific Style and Format for Authors, Editors, and Publishers*. 9th ed. University of Chicago Press.

Deming, Stephanie. 2009a. "Starting Off on the Right Foot." *Science Editor* 32 (3): 97–100.

Deming, Stephanie. 2009b. "Author-Friendly Onscreen Editing." *Science Editor* 32 (5): 169–70.

Deming, Stephanie. 2009c. "Author-Friendly Onscreen Editing: Part 2." *Science Editor* 32 (6): 203–4.

Deming, Stephanie. 2010a. "Some Prescriptions for Better Editor-Author Communication." *Science Editor* 33 (1): 25–26. https://www.csescienceeditor.org/article/between-author-and-editor-7/.

Deming, Stephanie. 2010b. "Queries: Conversing with the Author in Writing." *Science Editor* 33 (2): 59–60. https://www.csescienceeditor.org/article/author-editor-queries-conversing-author-writing/.

DeTora, Lisa, ed. 2020. *Regulatory Writing: An Overview*. 2nd ed. Regulatory Affairs Professionals Society.

DiAngelis, Heather. 2023. "Collaborative Copyediting: Helping the Author Help You." *Science Editor* 46 (4): e1–e2. https://www.csescienceeditor.org/article/collaborative-copyediting-helping-the-author-help-you/.

Document Design Project. 2014. *Guidelines for Document Designers*. American Institutes for Research. [reissued version of Felker et al., with new introduction.] https://cdn.ymaws.com/www.amwa.org/resource/resmgr/ResourcePage_/Guidelines.For.Document.Desi.pdf.

Einsohn, Amy, and Marilyn Schwartz. 2019. *The Copyeditor's Handbook: A Guide for Book Publishing and Corporate Communications*. 4th ed. University of California Press.

Faulkes, Zen. 2021. *Better Posters: Plan, Design, and Present an Academic Poster*. Pelagic.

Felker, Daniel B., Frances Pickering, Veda R. Charrow, V. Melissa Holland, and Janice C. Redish. 1981. *Guidelines for Document Designers*. American Institutes for Research. https://files.eric.ed.gov/fulltext/ED221866.pdf.

Fontanarosa, Phil B., Annette Flanagin, and Philip Greenland, eds. 2024. *Principles of Scientific Writing and Biomedical Publication: A JAMA Editors' Guide for Authors*. Oxford University Press. https://doi.org/10.1093/med/9780197783030.001.0001.

Gastel, Barbara. 1993. "Triage." *AMWA Journal* 8 (1): 26.

Gastel, Barbara. 2010. *Elements of Medical Terminology*. American Medical Writers Association.

Gastel, Barbara. 2011. "Satisfactions of Science Editing: Experienced Manuscript Editors Reflect." *Science Editor* 34 (2): 47–48. https://www.csescienceeditor.org/article/satisfactions-science-editing-experienced-manuscript-editors-reflect/.

Gastel, Barbara, and Robert A. Day. 2022. *How to Write and Publish a Scientific Paper*. 9th ed. Greenwood.

Grant, Maria J., and Andrew Booth. 2009. "A Typology of Reviews: An Analysis of 14 Review Types and Associated Methodologies." *Health Information and Libraries Journal* 26: 91–108. https://doi.org/10.1111/j.1471-1842.2009.00848.x.

Hamilton, Cindy W. 2012. *Tables and Graphs*. American Medical Writers Association.

Ibrahim, Andrew M. 2024. "Improving the Performance of Research Journals: Lessons Learned from the Visual Abstract." *Science Editor* 47 (2): 43–46.

https://www.csescienceeditor.org/article/improving-the-performance-of-research-journals/.

InterAcademy Partnership. 2016. *Doing Global Science: A Guide to Responsible Conduct in the Global Research Enterprise*. Princeton University Press. https://www.interacademies.org/publication/doing-global-science-guide-responsible-conduct-global-research-enterprise.

International Committee of Medical Journal Editors. [Updated] 2024. "Recommendations for the Conduct, Reporting, Editing, and Publication of Scholarly Work in Medical Journals." https://www.icmje.org/recommendations/.

International Committee of Medical Journal Editors. n.d. "Defining the Role of Authors and Contributors." https://www.icmje.org/recommendations/browse/roles-and-responsibilities/defining-the-role-of-authors-and-contributors.html.

Isaacson, Ruth A. 2023. "Text Recycling in Scientific Writing: What Editors Need to Know." *Science Editor* 46 (3): 107–9. https://www.csescienceeditor.org/article/text-recycling-in-scientific-writing/.

Jakubisin, Jenna. 2023. "Hiring and Thriving in the Remote Work Era." *Science Editor* 46 (4): 129–30. https://doi.org/10.36591/SE-D-4608-09.

Landis, Erin. 2023. "Remote Work Is a Trend with Staying Power: How Employees and Managers Can Succeed in This Brave New World." *Science Editor* 46 (1): 27–30. https://doi.org/10.36591/SE-D-4601-11.

Lang, Thomas A. 2010. *How to Write, Publish, and Present in the Health Sciences: A Guide for Clinicians and Laboratory Researchers*. American College of Physicians.

Lang, Thomas A., and Michelle Secic. 2006. *How to Report Statistics in Medicine: Annotated Guidelines for Authors, Editors, and Reviewers*. 2nd ed. American College of Physicians.

Lewis, Laurie. 2011. *What to Charge: Pricing Strategies for Freelancers and Consultants*. 2nd ed. Outskirts Press.

Loviglio, Lorraine. 1999. "A Day for the Red Book." *CBE Views* 22 (3): 91. https://csedev01.wpengine.com/wp-content/uploads/v22n3p91.pdf.

Mikel, Betsy. 2015. "25 Ways to Tighten Your Writing." https://collegesports communicators.com/news/2015/9/23/imported_0923154429.aspx.

National Center on Disability and Journalism. 2021. "Disability Language Style Guide." https://ncdj.org/style-guide/.

National Institutes of Health. 2025. "Biosketch Format Pages, Instructions and Samples." https://grants.nih.gov/grants-process/write-application/forms-directory/biosketch#biosketch-(non-fellowship):-biographical-sketch-format-page.

Office of Research Integrity. n.d. "Definition of Research Misconduct." https://ori.hhs.gov/definition-research-misconduct.

The Open Notebook. [2024.] "Guide to Using Alt-Text to Make Images More

Accessible." https://www.theopennotebook.com/guide-to-using-alt-text-to-make-images-more-accessible/.

Patrias, K. 2007–. *Citing Medicine: The NLM Style Guide for Authors, Editors, and Publishers*. 2nd ed. National Library of Medicine. https://www.ncbi.nlm.nih.gov/books/NBK7256/.

Purdue Online Writing Lab. n.d. "Style Guide Overview." https://owl.purdue.edu/owl/avoiding_plagiarism/guide_overview%20.html.

Riley, David S., Melissa S. Barber, Gunver S. Kienle, et al. 2017. "CARE Guidelines for Case Reports: Explanation and Elaboration Document." *Journal of Clinical Epidemiology* 18: 218–35. http://dx.doi.org/10.1016/j.jclinepi.2017.04.026.

Saller, Carol Fisher. 2016. *The Subversive Copy Editor: Advice from Chicago (or, How to Negotiate Good Relationships with Your Writers, Your Colleagues, and Yourself)*. 2nd ed. University of Chicago Press.

Scott, Jamie. 2019. "A Picture's Worth 1,000 Words: Disseminating Research Through Graphical and Visual Abstracts." *Science Editor* 42 (4): 142–43. https://www.csescienceeditor.org/article/a-pictures-worth-1000-words-disseminating-research-through-graphical-and-visual-abstracts/.

Sebastian, Felix, and Rachel Baron. 2024. "Artificial Intelligence: What the Future Holds for Multilingual Authors and Editing Professionals." *Science Editor* 47 (2): 38–42. https://doi.org/10.36591/SE-D-4702-01.

Semro, Madison. 2023a. "Editorial Fellowships: Acquainting Editorially Inclined Health Professionals and Scientists with the Workings of Journals." *Science Editor* 46 (1): 22–23. https://www.csescienceeditor.org/article/editorial-fellowships-health-professionals-scientists-workings-of-journals/.

Semro, Madison. 2023b. "Some Editorial Fellowship Programs in Science and Medicine." https://www.csescienceeditor.org/wp-content/uploads/2023/02/46-005-table.pdf.

Taylor, Robert B. 2018. *Medical Writing: A Guide for Clinicians, Educators, and Researchers*. Springer.

University of Chicago Press Editorial Staff. 2024. *The Chicago Manual of Style*. 18th ed. University of Chicago Press.

US Government Printing Office. 2016. *Style Manual: An Official Guide to the Form and Style of Federal Government Publications*. [31st ed.] US Government Printing Office. https://www.govinfo.gov/content/pkg/GPO-STYLEMANUAL-2016/pdf/GPO-STYLEMANUAL-2016.pdf.

Walshe, Catherine, Kim Beernart, Poh Heng Chong, Sonya Lowe, Sandra Martins Pereira, and Sarah Yardley. 2024. "Writing for the World: Enhancing Engagement and Connection with an International Audience." *Palliative Medicine* 38 (1): 4–6. https://doi.org/10.1177/02692163231215980.

Weiss, Edmond H. 2005. *The Elements of International English Style*. Sharpe.

Whalen, Elizabeth. 1992. "Keys to Success on Copyediting Tests." *CBE Views* 15 (3): 51–55.

World Health Organization. 2015. "World Health Organization Best Practices for the Naming of New Human Infectious Diseases." https://iris.who.int/bitstream/handle/10665/163636/WHO_HSE_FOS_15.1_eng.pdf?sequence=1.

Yin, Karen. 2024. *The Conscious Style Guide*. Little, Brown Spark.

Young, Roxanne K. 1997. "Ethical Dilemmas for Manuscript Editors." *CBE Views* 20 (1): 15–16. https://csedev01.wpengine.com/wp-content/uploads/v20n1p15-16.pdf.

Zeiger, Mimi. 2000. *Essentials of Writing Biomedical Research Papers*. 2nd ed. McGraw-Hill.

Index

abbreviations: conferences and, 147; copyediting and, 70–73, 88, 90, 92; lists of accepted, 14; resources for, 14–15, 19; substantive editing and, 104, 133

abstracts: conciseness and, 159; conferences and, 139–40, 143–44; copyediting and, 88, 99, 101, 103–5; exercises and, 137–38, 243–45; feedback and, 137–38, 243–45; final pass and, 57; graphical, 104; journal articles, 29, 88, 99, 101, 103–5, 115, 117–19, 122, 137, 140, 235; keywords and, 103–5; presentation, 6; PubMed and, 29; structured, 103–4, 115; style sheets and, 235–38; substantive editing and, 99, 101, 103–5, 115, 117–19, 122, 130, 137; visual, 104

Academic Phrasebank, 30

ACES: The Society for Editing, 23–24, 172, 224

acquisitions editors, 4–5, 46, 205, 229

acronyms: copyediting and, 64, 71–72; resources for, 19; style sheets and, 237, 240; substantive editing and, 122, 133

ACS [American Chemical Society] Guide to Scholarly Communication (Banik et al.), 14, 18

Adobe Acrobat, 31–32, 51, 171

Adobe Illustrator, 32

Adobe InDesign, 32

Adobe Photoshop, 32

adverbs, 68

ageism, 77–78

AI Sidequest (blog), 227

alt text, 91, 141–42, 145

AMA [American Medical Association] Manual of Style: AP style and, 18; author relationships and, 181; benefits of, 15–17; careers and, 213–14; copyediting and, 63–64, 70–82, 85–86, 89, 92; ethics and, 194, 196–97; exercises and, 241; manuscripts and, 15–16, 171; new editions of, 16–17; pitfalls and, 174, 181; proofreading and,

AMA [American Medical Association] Manual of Style (*continued*) 51, 171; quizzes of, 16, 20, 64, 89; as resource, 13–17, 20, 27, 34, 236; role of, 6; serial comma, 53; substantive editing and, 125
ambiguity, 44, 48, 68, 82, 152, 174, 206
American Association for the Advancement of Science, xiv
American Association of Dental Editors and Journalists (AADEJ), 23
American Cancer Society, 8
American Chemical Society (ACS), 14, 18
American Family Physician (journal), 28
American Heart Association, 8
American Medical Writers Association (AMWA): author relationships and, 175; careers and, 208, 211, 213, 219–20, 223, 227; certificates and, 219–21; copyediting and, 89; electronic tools and, 33; Engage and, 175; ethics and, 189–90, 197; freelancers and, 223–24; proofreading and, 51, 172; as resource, 19, 23–24, 26, 33, 51; style sheets and, 235, 237
American Psychological Association (APA) style, 17–18, 75, 86, 213
AMWA Journal, 24
anonymity, 91, 195
application essays: ambiguity and, 152; careers and, 21, 139, 149, 151–55, 158, 213; focus and, 153; ineffective beginning and, 153–54; ineffective ending and, 154; logic and, 153; mechanical errors and, 154–55; poor flow and, 153; readability and, 154; resources for, 21; support evidence and, 152–53; unsuitable length and, 154
ARRIVE (**A**nimal **R**esearch: **R**eporting of **I**n **V**ivo **E**xperiments), 123
artificial intelligence (AI): author lists and, 194; career effects of, 209, 213, 227–28; ChatGPT, 33; conciseness and, 72; ethics and, 194; non-native users of English and, 33; resources for, 33; screening by, 209, 213
Asian Council of Science Editors, 23
assistant editors, 4, 40, 208
assistive technologies, 78–79
Associação Brasileira de Editores Cientificos (Brazilian Association of Scientific Editors), 23
associate editors, 4, 23, 40, 233
Associated Press (AP) style: copyediting and, 71, 76, 85–86; resources for, 14, 18; substantive editing and, 124
Associated Press Stylebook, The (Associated Press), 14, 18, 76–77
Association of Health Care Journalists (AHCJ), 24, 184, 228
author lists, 38–39, 101–3, 156, 179, 193–94
author relationships: *AMA Manual of Style* and, 181; AMWA and, 175; author's editors and, 175–85; commissioning editors and, 181–84; communication and, 54–56, 177–78, 182–83; content and, 175, 177; context and, 179–80; copyediting and, 182; copyeditors and, 180; corrections and, 176–77, 183; courtesy and, 9–10, 12; credit and, 38, 178; CSE and, 184; early involvement and, 176; editing state and, 51–52; education and, 51–52, 180; ethics and, 178, 180, 191–96; expectations and, 177, 182; favoritism and, 189–90, 198; feedback and, 179; focus and, 178; freelancers and, 175,

181–83; funding sources and, 179; grammar and, 176; grant proposals and, 175–76, 179; handwritten notes to, 33–34; instructions to authors, 181; journal articles and, 102–3, 175, 178–79; logic and, 183; magazines and, 181; manuscripts and, 49–52, 175–84; news releases and, 181; overediting and, 177; permission and, 162; pre-submission editing and, 50, 55; promoting human connection and, 176–77; publication and, 180–81; punctuation and, 176, 178; qualities needed for, 176–78; queries and, 61–64, 176–81, 184; resources for, 184; respect and, 176, 188, 198; revisions and, 176–83; scientific papers and, 176, 180; style and, 181–82; submission and, 177, 179, 182; Track Changes and, 179, 181; websites and, 177, 179, 181, 251

author's editing, 52, 55, 179, 201, 213, 249

author's editors: author relationships and, 175–85; context and, 179; copyediting and, 61; cover notes and, 180; educational role and, 179–80; ethics and, 194–96, 200–201; exercises and, 247, 249; following up and, 180; grant proposals and, 8; journals and, 8; pitfalls and, 175; preferences and, 179; pre-submission editing and, 39, 42–43, 51, 55; proofreading and, 44, 170; revisions and, 46; role of, 8

Authors Without Borders (Bird, Hosseini, and Plemmons), 194

authorship: criteria, 38–39; ethics and, 38–39, 101–3, 156, 179, 193–94; substantive editing and, 102–3, 112, 115

autonomy, 188, 198

Avoiding Common Pitfalls in Medical Writing (Conners), 21

beneficence, 188, 198

bias, 6, 10, 76–79, 92, 190

billboard paragraph, 128–29

biosketches, 44, 134, 155, 157

biotechnology, 8, 28, 47, 204

Board of Editors in the Life Sciences (BELS), 24, 189–90, 220–21, 224; Code of Ethics, 189

book proposals, 4–5, 44–47, 96, 205

brand names, 75, 237

capitalization: careers and, 155–56; copyediting and, 63–64, 70–77, 87, 92; non-native users of English and, 168; proofreading and, 185; resources for, 15–16, 19; style sheets and, 237

captions: conciseness and, 161; conferences and, 143–44; copyediting and, 89–90; proofreading and, 171; substantive editing and, 129

CARE (**CA**se **RE**port) guidelines, 122

careers: acquisitions editors and, 205, 229; AI and, 209, 213, 227–28; *AMA Manual of Style* and, 213–14; AMWA and, 208, 211, 213, 219–20, 223, 227; APA style and, 213; application essays and, 21, 139, 149, 151–55, 158, 213; certificates and, 203, 213, 218–21, 231; Certified Medical Publication Professional, 221; choices in, xiii–xiv; clarity and, 150, 153, 156, 158; conciseness and, 150, 154, 156–57, 212, 220; conflicts of interest and, 222; consistency and, 152, 156, 158; content and, 149–54, 157, 205–6, 214, 221, 229–30; context and, 151, 155–56, 210, 216, 224;

careers (*continued*)
continuing education, 226–27; copyediting and, 149–50, 155, 204–8, 211, 213, 219, 229; cover letters, 209–12; CSE and, 208, 213, 224, 226–27; CVs, 46, 155–58, 209–14, 231; degrees and, 205, 210–14, 219–21; editing communications and, 149–58; Editorial Freelancers Association, 24, 223–24; editors-in-chief and, 204; education and, 155, 157, 204–6, 213, 219, 221; email discussion lists and, 22, 24–25, 31, 34, 175, 197, 224, 227; employment tests, 217–18; ethics and, 151, 220–21, 224; evaluation letters and, 149–51; feedback and, 151; focus and, 27, 151, 153, 155, 158, 211, 215–16, 220, 222–23, 227, 229; freelancers, 149, 204–11, 214, 217, 221–26, 231; grant proposals and, 157, 203–5; identifying openings, 208–9; instructions to authors and, 215; internships, 25, 27–28, 35, 209, 211, 214; interviews and, 214–17; IT and, 223; *JAMA*, 155; journal articles and, 155, 203, 211, 226–28; logic and, 153; magazines and, 211; maintaining motivation, 227–30; managing editors and, 204; manuscripts and, 157, 204–5, 211, 217–20, 223; mentors and, 11, 22, 25, 52, 92, 197, 207, 211, 213, 217, 220, 224, 242; news releases and, 204; NIH and, 157; nomination letters and, 139, 149–51, 158; office tools and, 31–34; organization and, 149, 155, 158, 220; personal skills and, 205–7; personal statements and, 151, 157; production editors and, 204; professional organizations and, 209, 211, 220, 226–27, 231; professional references and, 214; proofreading and, 209, 213, 219; publication and, 203–4, 221, 224, 230; publication lists and, 156–57; publishers and, 229–31; punctuation and, 150, 152, 156, 213, 220; queries and, 149–50, 218–19; range of settings for, 203–8; recommendation letters and, 21, 149–51, 158; remote work, 224–26; resources for, 22, 203–5, 208–10, 213, 215, 219–28; resumes and, 149, 155–58, 212–14, 231; science writing and, 210; scientific papers and, 151, 156; seeking positions, 208–17; specialists and, 150; style and, 156, 158, 213–14, 217, 225; submission and, 204–5; substantive editing and, 149–53, 204, 219, 229; websites and, 155, 157, 205, 208, 215, 222–24, 231

case description, 119

case reports: CARE and, 122; discussion and, 120; ethics and, 195; IMRAD format and, 121; introduction and, 119; resources for, 21; role of, 118–19; substantive editing and, 95–97, 116, 118–22, 135; written permission for, 119

Center for Plain Language, 163

Centers for Disease Control and Prevention (CDC), 8, 28, 66, 71, 163

certificates: AMWA, 219–20; careers and, 203, 213, 218–21, 231; degrees and, 25–26, 35, 213, 219–21; resources for, 19, 22, 24–26, 35; University of California, San Diego, 26; University of Chicago, 26

certification: BELS and, 220; careers and, 203, 213, 218–21, 231; MWC credential, 220–21; resources for, 24, 31

Certified Medical Publication Professional (CMPP), 221
Chartered Institute of Editing and Proofreading, 27
ChatGPT, 33
Chicago Guide for Freelance Editors, The (Brenner), 21, 222
Chicago Manual of Style, The (University of Chicago Press Editorial Staff): benefits of, 17–18; copyediting and, 76; proofreading and, 171–72; as resource, 14, 17–18, 51, 76, 171–72
Chinese Medical Association, xiv
chromosomes, 17
citations, 16, 86, 114–15, 147, 192
clarity: ambiguity and, 44, 48, 68, 82, 152, 174, 206; careers and, 150, 153, 156, 158; conciseness and, 161–62; copyediting and, 72; CVs and, 156; exercises and, 244; importance of, 9, 12; lack of, 32; non-native users of English and, 169; pitfalls in, 173; proofreading and, 171; substantive editing and, 104, 112, 127, 133, 135; visibility and, 31, 49, 57, 171
Clinical Chemistry (journal), 30, 89
colons, 67, 101, 236
commas: copyediting and, 53, 65–67, 80, 85–88; nonrestrictive clauses and, 52, 65–66; proofreading and, 172; resources for, 14, 17–18. *See also* serial commas
commissioning editors, 181–84
completeness: importance of, 9–10, 12; screening and, 40; substantive editing and, 96–97, 135
compound modifiers, 67–68
compound sentences, 65
conciseness: abstracts and, 159; ambiguity and, 44, 48, 68, 82, 152, 174, 206; AI and, 72; captions and, 161; careers and, 150, 154, 156–57, 212, 220; clarity and, 161–62; condensing wordy phrases, 160; conferences and, 145; context and, 161; copyediting and, 159; CVs and, 156; double negatives and, 161; elaboration and, 48, 57, 122, 130; exercises and, 185, 244–45; general readership and, 160; grant proposals and, 159; importance of, 9–10, 12; logic and, 6, 50; manuscripts and, 159–62; needless words and, 159–60; nouns and, 160–61, 184; overediting and, 173; passive voice and, 161; queries and, 161–62; readability and, 184; scientific papers and, 162; substantive editing and, 104, 127; verbs and, 160–61, 184
conferences: abbreviations and, 147; abstracts and, 139–40, 143–44; alt text and, 141–42, 145; analogous works and, 145–48; captions and, 143–44; conciseness and, 145; consistency and, 147; content and, 139–48; context and, 139–41, 146–47; contributors and, 147–48; copyediting and, 139; credit and, 141, 143; editing communications and, 139–48, 158; feedback and, 147; focus and, 139; format and, 141, 143–44, 146–47; grant proposals and, 139; IMRAD and, 143; instructions to authors and, 146–47; journal articles and, 140; logic and, 140; manuscripts and, 142, 146; non-native users of English and, 141; organization and, 140, 146; parallelism and, 141; poster presentations, 142–45, 158; proceedings and, 139, 145–48, 158; professional organizations and, 22–24; proofreading and, 148; publishers and, 147;

conferences (*continued*)
resources for, 16, 22–24, 33, 142, 146; revisions and, 141, 146–48; role of, 5; scientific papers and, 143; slide presentations, 140–42, 158; style and, 140, 146–48; submission and, 146; substantive editing and, 123, 125, 139, 146; webinars and, 22–23, 25, 33, 172, 226–28; websites and, 141
confidants, 49
confidence intervals, 81, 109
confidentiality, 42, 96, 188–89, 195–98, 249
conflicts of interest: careers and, 222; ethics and, 96, 126, 188, 190, 195–200, 222, 246; substantive editing and, 96, 126; transparency and, 190
conjunctions, 65–66
Conners, Deanna Erin, 21
connotation, 48–49, 57, 60, 77
Conscious Style Guide, The (Yin), 76
consistency: conferences and, 147; copyediting and, 54, 77, 88–89, 92; pre-submission editing and, 43, 50; proofreading and, 172; resources for, 19; role of, 6, 9–10, 12; substantive editing and, 99, 101, 107, 132–34; variation vs., 48, 57
CONSORT (**CON**solidated **S**tandards **O**f **R**eporting **T**rials), 101, 122
content: author relationships and, 175, 177; author's editors and, 39; careers and, 149–54, 157, 205–6, 214, 221, 229–30; conferences and, 139–48; copyediting and, 53–54, 61, 69, 79–80, 89–91; ethics and, 187–93; exercises and, 244; focus and, 4, 20, 24, 42, 54, 69, 91, 96, 139, 153, 189; non-native users of English and, 169; organization and, 7, 50, 53–54, 57, 61, 95–96, 134–35, 137, 140, 146, 149; peer review and, 40, 42; pre-submission editing and, 49–50; proofreading and, 172; readability and, 162–63; resources for, 15, 17–20, 23–24, 30; substantive editing and, 95–104, 107–9, 115–17, 121–22, 125–26, 128–29, 132–37; types of, 3–11
context: author relationships and, 179–80; author's editors and, 55; careers and, 151, 155–56, 210, 216, 224; conciseness and, 161; conferences and, 139–41, 146–47; copyediting and, 64, 68, 71–74, 80, 84, 91; ethics and, 195–96; exercises and, 242–43; internships and, 27; journal articles and, 37, 116, 119, 155, 196, 242; medical editors and, 11; style and, 18, 55, 71, 84, 116; substantive editing and, 101, 104–5, 109–11, 114–16, 119–22, 126, 130, 135, 137; understanding, 37–38
continuing medical education (CME), xvi, 72
contributors: authors and, 103; conferences and, 147–48; CRediT and, 103; ethics and, 194; substantive editing and, 102–3, 134
COPE (Committee on Publication Ethics), 30, 196–97
copyediting: abbreviations and, 70–73, 88, 90, 92; abstracts and, 88, 99, 101, 103–5; acronyms and, 64, 71–72; alt text and, 91; *AMA Manual of Style* and, 63–64, 70–82, 85–86, 89, 92; AMWA and, 89; AP style and, 71, 76, 85–86; APA style and, 75, 86; author relationships and, 182; author's editors and, 61; beyond, 91; capitalization and, 63–64,

70–77, 87, 92; captions and, 89–90; careers and, 149–50, 155, 204, 206, 213, 219; CDC and, 66, 71; clarity and, 72; colons, 67, 101, 236; commas, 65–67, 80, 85–88; commonly confused terms, 73–74; conciseness and, 159; conferences and, 139; conformity with publication's style, 84–88; consistency and, 77, 88–89, 92; content and, 61, 69, 79–80, 89–91; context and, 64, 68, 71–74, 80, 84, 91; corrections and, 59–64, 68, 89; credit and, 90; *The CSE Manual* and, 75–77, 79, 81; dictionaries and, 70, 73; DOIs and, 87; education and, 63; eponyms, 75–76; ethics and, 62; exercises and, 92–93, 241–42; fact-checking and, 91; feature articles and, 77; feedback and, 92; figures, 87–91; format and, 59, 75, 79, 86–90, 92; freelancers and, 68; general readership and, 86, 88; grammar and, 59, 64, 68–73, 90, 92; grant proposals and, 67, 74–75, 89; hyphens and, 67–68; importance of, 59–60, 91–92; indicating edits, 60–61; instructions to authors, 71, 87–89; journal articles, 67, 74–75, 78, 80–81, 88–91; legends and, 90; logic and, 61; magazines and, 67, 91; manuscripts, 63–68, 72, 76, 84, 87–91; marks, 60; mechanical errors and, 59–84, 92; medical word usage and, 73–76; mentors and, 92; news releases and, 85; NIH and, 66, 71; nomenclature and, 74–75; nonrestrictive clauses, 52, 65–66; nouns, 67–71, 78–79, 83–84, 87; numbers, 62, 64, 67, 79–82, 85, 86, 88, 90; organization and, 61; parallelism and, 69; peer review and, 62, 80; permissions and, 90, 98; plagiarism and, 62; plurals, 16, 70, 92; proofreading and, 88; publication and, 59–60, 65, 67, 76, 88; publishers and, 68, 75; punctuation and, 59, 64–70, 85–87, 90, 92; queries and, 59–64, 80–82, 89–91; resources for, 16, 19–20, 31, 34, 60, 76, 87, 91, 184; respect and, 76–79, 92; revisions and, 59–61, 82–83; role of, 5–8, 59; scientific papers, 74; semicolons, 66–67; serial commas, 85, 88; specialists and, 83; spelling, 60–64, 70–73, 79, 85, 90, 92; stacked nouns, 84; statistics, 64, 79–82, 92; style and, 59–67, 70–92; submission and, 90, 96, 103, 112, 116, 134; substantive editing and, 95, 99, 113, 120–21, 130; syntax, 82–84, 220; tables, 87–91; tagging, 91; toponyms, 75–76; Track Changes, 60–61; websites and, 86, 89; word usage, 59, 64, 73–79, 92

Copyediting-L, 31

copyeditors: author relationships and, 180; careers and, 204–5, 208, 211, 229; resources for, 19–20, 34; role of, 5, 7–8, 59–60, 71, 77–84, 87–91; style sheets and, 236, 239; substantive editing and, 96, 113

Copyeditor's Handbook, The (Einsohn and Schwartz), 19–20, 34, 60, 64

Copyeditors' Knowledge Base, 31

Copyeditor's Workbook, The (Bűky, Schwartz, and Einsohn), 20

corrections: author relationships and, 176–77, 183; copyediting and, 59–64, 68, 89; ethics and, 187, 194, 201; grammar, 1, 9, 11, 32, 53, 68, 154, 168, 176; importance of, 4; mechanical errors, 53, 60–84,

corrections (*continued*)
201, 250; non-native users of English and, 169; proofreading and, 51, 170–71; resources for, 32; revisions and, 52–53, 60; spelling, 5, 9, 29, 53, 60–61, 95, 170; syntax, 82–84, 220; word usage, 5, 9

correctness, 9–10, 12, 173

corresponding author, 39, 44, 156

Council of Asian Science Editors, 23

Council of Biology Editors, 189

Council of Science Editors (CSE): author relationships and, 184; careers and, 208, 213, 224, 226–27; copyediting and, 75–76, 81; *The CSE Manual*, 13–14, 17–18, 22–24, 75–77, 79, 81, 196, 213; ethics and, 189, 194–97; pitfalls and, 175; *Recommendations for Promoting Integrity in Scientific Journal Publications*, 22, 194, 196, 197; resources of, 13–14, 17, 22–23, 33

courtesy, 9–10, 12

cover letters, 39, 46, 166, 209–12, 231

cover notes, 52, 146, 180

COVID-19 pandemic, 16, 72, 119, 206, 228, 240

credit: author relationships and, 178; authorship and, 38–39, 102–3, 112, 115, 193–94, 199, 250; conferences and, 141, 143; contributor roles and, 103; copyediting and, 90; ethics and, 194; funding sources and, 113; for medical editors, 4; online courses and, 27; senior researcher and, 38

CRediT (Contributor Role Taxonomy), 103

cross-references, 171

cucumber science (salami science), 193, 199

curriculum vitae (CVs), 212–14; biosketches and, 44, 134, 155, 157; book proposals and, 46; careers and, 46, 149, 155–58, 209–14, 231; clarity and, 156; conciseness and, 156; description of, 155; length of, 155; publication history and, 29, 155; publication lists and, 155–57; telling your story with, 210

Day, Robert A., 21

dead copy, 172

deck, 164

degrees: bachelor's, 3, 25–26, 210, 213, 220–21; careers and, 205, 210–14, 219–21; certificates and, 25–26, 35, 213, 219–21; resources for, 26–27, 32, 35; role of, 1, 3

Deming, Stephanie, 61, 64, 177, 184

denotation, 48–49, 57

desk reject, 42

dictionaries: copyediting and, 70, 73; as resource, 18–19, 28–29, 34; style sheets and, 147, 236, 239

Disability Language Style Guide (National Center on Disability and Journalism), 77

Doing Global Science (InterAcademy Partnership), 196

DOIs (digital object identifiers), 87

Dorland's Illustrated Medical Dictionary, 18–19

double negatives, 161

Dragonfly Editorial, 31

Drug Information Association (DIA), 23–24

drugs: approval of, 6, 205–6; brand, 75, 237; FDA and, 6, 47; generic, 75, 237; pharmaceuticals and, 8, 17, 20, 28, 47, 161, 204–6, 211; recommended dosage, 81; resources for, 29; side effects and, 67, 101, 110, 126; substantive editing and, 101, 107, 119, 125, 250

duplicate publication, 193, 199

Editorial Freelancers Association (EFA), 24, 27, 172, 221–24
editors-in-chief: careers and, 204; ethics and, 198; exercises and, 247; role of, 4–5, 8, 40–41
education: author relationships and, 51–52, 180; careers and, 155, 157, 204–6, 213, 219, 221; continuing medical education, xvi, 72; copyediting and, 63; email discussion lists, 22, 24–25, 31, 34, 175, 197, 224, 227; ethics and, 191, 195–96; internships, 25, 27–28, 35, 209, 211, 214; MOOCs, 27, 228; online forums, 22, 31, 34, 175, 197, 224, 227; opportunities in, 25–28; patient, 7; periodicals and, 18, 22, 26, 33, 87, 184, 224; quizzes, 16, 20, 64, 89; resources for, 13, 16, 19, 24–28, 31, 35; substantive editing and, 98, 119, 123, 130, 134; webinars, 22–23, 25, 33, 172, 226–28
educational editing, 51–52, 63, 180
elaboration, 48, 57, 122, 130
electronic format, 90, 171
Elements of International English Style, The (Weiss), 169
Elements of Medical Terminology (Gastel), 19
Elsevier, 196
em dashes, 67
email addresses, 212
email discussion lists: careers and, 22, 24–25, 31, 34, 175, 197, 224, 227; ethics and, 197, 224; resources for, 22, 24–25, 31, 34
en dashes, 67
EndNote, 33
eponyms, 75–76
EQUATOR (**E**nhancing the **QUA**lity and **T**ransparency **O**f health **R**esearch), 30, 121–23, 135
Essentials of Writing Biomedical Research Papers (Zeiger), 21
"Ethical and Legal Considerations" (*AMA Manual of Style*), 197
ethics: AI and, 194; *AMA Manual of Style* and, 194, 196–97; AMWA and, 189–90, 197; ARRIVE and, 123; author relationships and, 178, 180, 191–96; author's editors and, 194–96, 200–201; authorship and, 38–39, 101–3, 156, 179, 193–94; autonomy and, 188, 198; beneficence and, 188, 198; Board of Editors in the Life Sciences Code of Ethics, 189; careers and, 151, 220–21, 224; case reports and, 195; certificates and, 190, 200; confidentiality and, 42, 96, 188–89, 195–98, 249; conflicts of interest and, 96, 126, 188, 190, 195–200, 222, 246; content and, 187–93; context and, 195–96; contributors and, 194; COPE and, 30–31, 196–97; copyediting and, 62; corrections and, 187, 194, 201; credit and, 194; CSE and, 189, 194–97; cucumber science and, 193; duplicate publication, 193, 199; editors-in-chief and, 198; education and, 191, 195–96; email discussion lists and, 197, 224; exercises and, 199–201, 245–51; fabrication and, 192, 199; falsification and, 192, 199; favoritism and, 189–90, 198; feedback and, 191; focus and, 189; freelancers and, 189–90, 201; funding sources and, 188, 195; ghost authors and, 194; grant proposals and, 189, 199–200; guest authors and, 194; integrity and, 189–98; journal articles and, 190, 196, 201; justice, 188, 198; manuscripts and, 189–

ethics (*continued*)
92, 195, 198–201; mechanical errors and, 201; mentors and, 197; news releases and, 190, 200; nonmaleficence and, 188, 198; obligations of, 189–91; Office of Research Integrity, 192; organization and, 201; overstatement and, 190–91, 199–200, 248; peer review and, 192, 195–96, 200–201; permissions and, 98, 189, 195, 249; plagiarism and, 32, 62, 166, 192–93, 199; professional organizations and, 197, 224; publication, 180, 187, 190–99; publishers and, 196; queries and, 191, 199; rationality, 188, 198; resources for, 14–16, 19, 30, 189–97; revisions and, 191; role of, 6; salami science and, 193, 199; scientific papers and, 196; style and, 192–97, 201; submission and, 192–95; substantive editing and, 96, 98, 127, 135; text recycling and, 193; transparency, 111, 188, 190, 195, 198, 245; underlying principles for, 187–89; universalizability, 188, 198; veracity and, 187, 198; websites and, 194, 196
European Association of Science Editors (EASE), 23–24, 227
European Science Editing (journal), 23
evaluation letters, 149–51
Everyday Words for Public Health Communication (CDC), 163
Excel, 31

fabrication, 192, 199
Facebook, 31
fact-checking, 91
falsification, 192, 199
favoritism, 189–90, 198
feature articles, 77, 127–29
feedback: abstracts and, 137–38, 243–45; author relationships and, 179; careers and, 151; conferences and, 147; copyediting and, 92; ethics and, 191; exercises and, 243–45, 249; peer review and, 40, 45–46; substantive editing and, 112, 137–38
figures, 88–91
final approval, 41, 102
focus: application essays and, 153; author relationships and, 178; careers and, 27, 151, 153, 155, 158, 211, 215–16, 220, 222–23, 227, 229; conferences and, 139; content and, 4, 20, 24, 42, 54, 69, 91, 96, 139, 153, 189; ethics and, 189; exercises and, 244; guidance and, 6, 78, 95, 127, 139, 166; non-native users of English and, 166, 168; readership and, 39; substantive editing and, 96–97, 101, 109–12, 117–20, 126–30, 133, 135
Fogarty, Mignon, 227
Food and Drug Administration (FDA), 6, 47
format: careers and, 156–58, 214; conferences and, 141, 143–44, 146–47; consistent, 10, 90, 132, 141, 146, 156–57, 213–14; copyediting and, 59, 75, 79, 86–90, 92; electronic, 90, 171; IMRAD, 99–101, 103, 114–18, 121, 135, 143; inverted pyramid, 124–25, 127; pitfalls and, 175; pre-submission editing and, 39; proofreading and, 171; publishers and, 2, 6, 14, 22, 51, 171; readability and, 164; required, 1–2, 6–7, 39, 43, 47, 50, 87, 90, 144, 157; resources for, 14, 22, 33; role of, 1–2; style and, 1–2, 6–7, 14, 22, 41, 43, 51, 55, 59–61, 71, 75, 86–88, 92, 116, 121, 124–25, 146–47, 156,

170, 196; substantive editing and, 99, 101, 103–4, 109, 114–18, 121, 124–27, 132, 135
freelancers, 249–51; AMWA and, 223–24; author relationships and, 175, 181–83; careers and, 149, 204–11, 214, 217, 221–26, 231; *The Chicago Guide for Freelance Editors*, 222; considerations for, 221–24; copyediting and, 68; Editorial Freelancers Association, 24, 27, 172, 221–24; ethics and, 189–90, 201; gradual transition to, 223; payment of, 22, 174, 223; proofreading and, 172; remote work and, 224–26; resources for, 21–24, 27, 31, 34, 223–24; role of, 1, 5, 8–9, 12; substantive editing and, 96, 123, 130
funding sources: author relationships and, 179; credit and, 113; ethics and, 188, 195; mission of, 45; substantive editing and, 113, 115, 130–32; transparency and, 245

Gastel, Barbara, 19, 21, 162
general readership: careers and, 228, 230; conciseness and, 160; copyediting and, 86, 88; journal articles and, 123–30; materials for, 1, 12, 14, 18, 21, 24, 29–30, 44, 47, 163, 169; readability and, 163–64; resources for, 14, 18, 21, 24, 29–30; style sheets and, 239–40; substantive editing and, 123–29, 135
generic drugs, 75, 237
genes, 17, 74, 84
ghost authors, 194
glossaries, 15, 164
Google Docs, 31
grammar: adverbs, 68; articles, 167; author relationships and, 176; careers and, 150–56, 220, 227; checkers for, 32, 154, 168; conjunctions, 65–66; copyediting and, 59, 64, 68–73, 90, 92; corrections of, 1, 9, 11, 32, 53, 68, 154, 168, 176; double negatives, 161; mechanical errors, 64, 68–73, 90, 92; non-native users of English, 168–69; nouns, 32, 67–71, 78–79, 83–84, 87, 156, 160–61, 172, 184; parallelism and, 69, 141, 156, 158, 213; pitfalls and, 174; prepositions, 69, 162, 167–68, 185; proofreading and, 170–71; resources for, 15–16, 19, 27, 30, 32; role of, 1, 5, 9, 11; stereotypical editor and, 1; substantive editing and, 95, 127; verbs, 32, 51, 66, 68–69, 160–61, 168, 184–85, 236
Grammar Girl, 227
Grammarly, 32
grant proposals: author relationships and, 175–76, 179; author's editors and, 8; careers and, 157, 203–5; conciseness and, 159; conferences and, 139; copyediting and, 67, 74–75, 89; deadlines for, 45; ethics and, 189, 199–200; exercises and, 245, 248; funding and, 2, 6, 45, 74, 130, 134–35, 157, 180; journal articles and, 1–2, 6, 8, 12, 21, 26–27, 37, 44, 50, 67, 74–75, 89, 95–96, 133–34, 155, 171, 175, 179, 203; NIH and, 44–45, 66, 157; preparation of, 21, 44–45; pre-submission editing, 50; principal investigators and, 45, 134; proofreading and, 171; resources for, 21, 23, 26–27; role of, 1–2, 6, 8, 12; specific aims and, 130–31; study sections and, 45; style and, 67, 75, 96, 134; substantive editing and, 95–96, 130–35
graphical abstracts, 104, 115, 137
guest authors, 194

Guide to Scientific Writing (Annesley and Derish), 30
Guidelines for Document Designers (Document Design Project), 163

Health Insurance Portability and Accountability Act (HIPAA), 71, 241
heavy editing, 53, 57
How to Report Statistics in Medicine (Lang and Secic), 21, 82
How to Write and Publish a Scientific Paper (Gastel and Day), 21, 162
How to Write, Publish, and Present in the Health Sciences (Lang), 21
hyphens: compound modifiers and, 67–68; copyediting and, 67–68; resources for, 16, 19, 24; style sheets and, 237

IMRAD (introduction, methods, results, and discussion) format: conferences and, 143; review articles and, 116, 118; substantive editing and, 99–101, 103, 114–18, 121, 135
indexes: *The Chicago Manual of Style* and, 14; *The CSE Manual* and, 14; editing back matter, 148; production editors and, 5; style manuals and, 14–15; substantive editing and, 105
information technology (IT), 223
institutional animal care and use committee (IACUC), 107, 192
institutional review board (IRB), 107, 192
instructions to authors: author relationships and, 181; careers and, 215; conferences and, 146–47; copyediting and, 71, 87–89; resources for, 30, 34; style sheets and, 236; substantive editing and, 105
Instructions to Authors in the Health Sciences (website), 30
integrity: ethics and, 189–98; Office of Research Integrity, 192; *Recommendations for Promoting Integrity in Scientific Journal Publications*, 22, 194, 196–97; resources for, 22, 194, 196; substantive editing and, 102
InterAcademy Partnership, 196
International Academy of Nursing Editors (INANE), 23
International Committee of Medical Journal Editors (ICMJE), 38, 102, 194–97
International Society for Medical Publication Professionals (ISMPP), 23–25, 221
internships, 25, 27–28, 35, 209, 211, 214
interviews, 214–17
inverted pyramid format, 124–25, 127
invisibility, 49, 57
iThenticate, 32

JAMA (*Journal of the American Medical Association*), 28–29, 155
job announcements, 22, 208, 210, 213
journal articles: abstracts, 29, 88, 99, 101, 103–4, 115–19, 122, 137, 140, 235; acknowledgments, 112–13; author relationships and, 102–3, 175, 178–79; careers and, 155, 203, 211, 226–28; case reports, 118–21; conferences and, 140; context and, 37, 116, 119, 155, 196, 242; copyediting and, 67, 74–75, 78, 80–81, 88–91; discussion, 109–12; editorial involvement in, 40–41; ethics and, 190, 196, 201; exercises and, 135–37, 242–43, 248; grant proposals and, 1–2, 6, 8, 12, 21, 26–27, 37, 44, 50, 67, 74–75, 89, 95–96, 133–34, 155, 171, 175,

179, 203; guidelines for, 121–23; importance of, 38; International Committee of Medical Journal Editors and, 38, 102, 194, 196–97; introduction, 105–6; keywords and, 103–5, 127; methods section, 106–8; non-native users of English and, 165, 169; organization of, 242–43; peer review and, 2, 23, 40, 42, 45, 50, 80, 111, 195–96, 201, 248–49; proofreading and, 170; references, 113–14; rejection and, 39–43, 50, 181; reporting research, 99–115; resources for, 13, 15, 20–21, 24–34; results section, 108–9; review, 116–18; revisions and, 37, 40–41, 101; scope of editorial work in, 1, 6–12; screening, 39–42, 46, 136, 208–9, 242; style sheets and, 235; submission of, 4–5, 8, 38–39, 43–44, 50, 90, 96, 103, 116, 170, 172, 179, 192–95, 204–5; substantive editing and, 95–96, 99–127, 133–37; title, 101–2
Journal of General Internal Medicine, 28
Journal of Young Investigators, The, 26
justice, 188, 198

keywords: abstracts and, 103–5; careers and, 209, 213; journal articles, 103–4, 127; substantive editing and, 103–5, 127
Knight Science Journalism Program, MIT, 26
Korean Council of Science Editors, 23

Lang, Thomas A., 21, 82
legends, 90
levels of editing, 52–55
Lewis, Laurie, 22, 223
liberal arts, 1, 9, 25
light editing, 53
literary editing, 48–49
live copy, 172
logic: application essays and, 153; author relationships and, 183; careers and, 153; conciseness and, 6, 50; conferences and, 140; copyediting and, 50, 61; readability and, 164; substantive editing and, 1, 96–98, 106, 111, 117, 135

macroediting, 53–54, 57
magazines: author relationships and, 181; careers and, 211; copyediting and, 47, 67, 91; editors-in-chief of, 4–5; readability and, 164; resources for, 26; role of, 4–8; substantive editing and, 123–24
managing editors, 5, 8, 40–41, 204
manuscript editors: author relationships and, 175, 178, 182; careers and, 211; conferences and, 146; copyediting and, 43, 91; ethics and, 189, 191–92, 198–200; exercises and, 246; proofreading and, 170; as resource, 15–16, 23; role of, 5–9; style sheets and, 235
manuscripts: acquisitions editors and, 4–5; *AMA Manual of Style* and, 15–16, 171; author relationships and, 175–84; careers and, 157, 204–5, 211, 217–20, 223; conciseness and, 159–62; conferences and, 142, 146; copyediting and, 43, 63–68, 72, 76, 84, 87–91; ethics and, 189–92, 195, 198–201; exercises and, 246–47, 249–50; managing editors and, 5; non-native users of English and, 166–69; pitfalls and, 173–75; production editors and, 5; proofreading and, 170–72; refining, 8; resources for, 15–23, 29–33; submission of, 39, 46, 51; substantive editing and, 96, 99–100, 103, 106, 109–14; tagging, 91

massive open online courses (MOOCs), 27, 228
MD Anderson Cancer Center, 28, 61, 184
mechanical errors: application essays and, 154–55; capitalization and, 63–64, 70–77, 87, 92; common, 60–84; copyediting and, 53–54, 59, 60–84; corrections of, 53, 60–84, 201, 250; ethics and, 201; exercises and, 250; figures and, 88–91; grammar and, 64, 68–73, 90, 92; plurals, 16, 70, 92; proofreading and, 51, 170, 185; punctuation, 64–70, 85–87, 90, 92; spacing, 51, 57, 87, 157, 168, 170–71; spelling, 61, 63–64, 70–73, 79, 85, 90, 92; style and, 51, 53–54, 60, 65, 170, 201, 250; tables and, 88–91
medical devices, 6, 8, 47, 199–200, 246
medical editors: author relationships and, 11, 175–84; conciseness and, 159–62; credit for, 4; ethics and, 187–201; as helping profession, 2; importance of, 2; non-native users of English and, 165–69; overview, 3–11; pharmaceuticals and, 8; pitfalls in, 173–75; preparation by, 37–58; readability and, 162–65; resources for, 13–36; role of, 1–12; style sheets and, 235–40. *See also* copyediting; proofreading; substantive editing
Medical Editors (Facebook group), 31
Medical Writer Certified (MWC), 220–21
Medical Writing (Taylor), 21
medium editing, 53–54
MedlinePlus, 29–30, 100
Mendeley, 33
mentors: careers and, 11, 22, 25, 52, 92, 197, 207, 211, 213, 217, 220, 224, 242; copyediting and, 92; ethics and, 197; resources for, 11, 22, 25
Merck Manuals, 20
Merriam-Webster's Collegiate Dictionary, 19
microediting, 53–54, 57
Microsoft Teams, 215
Microsoft Word, 31–32, 80, 85, 164, 171–72
MIT, 26
Mulford Health Science Library, University of Toledo, 30
multi-language authors, 165

National Association of Science Writers (NASW), 23–24, 184, 228
National Center for Health Care Technology, xiv
National Center on Disability and Journalism, 77
National Institutes of Health (NIH), xiv; BIOART and, 32; careers and, 157; copyediting and, 66, 71; exercises and, 242; grants and, 44–45, 66, 157; resources of, 29, 32, 44–45; as single entity, 66; style sheets and, 240; substantive editing and, 100
National Library of Medicine, 29, 156
native English speakers, 4, 68, 167–69
New England Journal of Medicine, 28–29
news releases: author relationships and, 181; careers and, 204; copyediting and, 38, 85; ethics and, 190, 200; exercises and, 247–48; general readership and, 123–27; journal articles and, 123–27; resources for, 14, 18; role of, 7–8; substantive editing and, 123–29, 135
news stories: copyediting and, 38; inverted pyramid format and,

124–25, 127; public information officers and, 126; resources for, 18; substantive editing and, 123–29; summary leads and, 124
newsletters, 7–8, 24, 124, 181, 214
newspapers, 7, 18, 26, 85, 123, 205, 210, 226
Newsweek (magazine), xiv
No Markup setting, 57
nomenclature, 10, 14–15, 18, 74–75
nomination letters, 139, 149–51, 158
nonmaleficence, 188, 198
non-native users of English: AI and, 33; capitalization and, 168; clarity and, 169; conferences and, 141; corrections and, 169; cultural differences and, 165–66; grammar and, 168–69; journal articles and, 165, 169; linguistics and, 167–69; manuscripts and, 166–69; multi-language authors and, 165; native speakers and, 4, 68, 167–69; respect and, 165
nonrestrictive clauses, 52, 65–66
nouns: conciseness and, 160–61, 184; copyediting and, 67–71, 78–79, 83–84, 87; derived from verbs, 160–61; pronouns, 70, 79, 83, 172; proper, 156; resources for, 32; stacked, 84
numbers: confidence intervals, 81, 109; copyediting and, 62, 64, 67, 79–82, 85, 86, 88, 90; implausible, 10; queries and, 62; resources for, 14–15, 17; style and, 86, 236; writing, 14, 85
nurses, 19, 23, 105, 136, 185
nut graf, 128–29

Office of Research Integrity, 192
O'Moore-Klopf, Katharine, 31
On Being a Scientist (Committee on Science, Engineering, and Public Policy), 196
One-Look Dictionary Search, 19, 28–29
online resources: careers and, 203–5, 209–10, 215, 219, 224–28; conferences and, 142, 146; copyediting and, 60, 76, 87, 91; ethics and, 196–97; Facebook, 31; forums, 22, 31, 34, 175, 197, 224, 227; MOOCs, 27, 228; pitfalls in, 175; proofreading and, 170–72; substantive editing and, 137; use of, 13–31, 34–35
Online Writing Lab (OWL), Purdue University, 14, 30
organization: content and, 7, 50, 53–54, 57, 61, 95–96, 134–35, 137, 140, 146, 149; copyediting and, 53–54, 57; ethics and, 201; exercises and, 242–43, 250; managing editors and, 5; production editors and, 5; role of, 1, 5, 7; substantive editing and, 1, 61, 95–97, 108, 132, 134–37
organizations, professional: careers and, 209, 211, 220, 226–27, 231; conferences and, 22–24; email discussion lists and, 22, 24–25, 31, 34, 175, 197, 224, 227; ethics and, 197, 224; job announcements and, 22, 208, 210, 213; online forums and, 22, 31, 34, 175, 197, 224, 227; periodicals and, 18, 22, 26, 33, 87, 184, 224; resources of, 13, 22–25, 31, 35; webinars and, 22–23, 25, 33, 172, 226–28
orphans, 171
overediting, 159, 173–75, 177, 218
overstatement, 190–91, 199–200, 248

Pan American Health Organization, 8
parallelism, 69, 141, 156, 158, 213
passive voice, 161
PDF (portable document format) files, 32, 44, 51, 171

peer review: careers and, 229; copyediting and, 62, 80; ethics and, 192, 195–96, 200–201; exercises and, 247–49; grant proposals and, 45; journal articles and, 2, 23, 40, 42, 45, 50, 80, 111, 195–96, 201, 248–49; referees and, 42; resources for, 23; role of, 2, 5; substantive editing and, 99, 111, 130–31
Peking University Health Center, xiv
PerfectIt, 32
periodicals, 18, 22, 26, 33, 87, 184, 224
Perkins, Maxwell, 49
permissions: copyediting and, 90, 98; ethics and, 98, 189, 195, 249; exercises and, 249; plagiarism and, 32; substantive editing and, 98, 119
personal statements, 151, 157
pharmaceuticals: biotechnology and, 8, 28, 47, 204; conciseness and, 161; drugs and, 8, 17, 20, 28, 47, 161, 204–6, 211; medical editors and, 8; side effects and, 67, 101, 110, 126
pharmacokinetics, 250
physicians: role of medical editing and, 2–3, 6; substantive editing and, 120, 128
pitches, 47, 181
pitfalls: *AMA Manual of Style* and, 174, 181; clarity and, 173; CSE and, 175; format and, 175; grammar and, 174; overediting, 159, 173–75, 177, 218; punctuation and, 174; queries and, 175; style and, 174
plagiarism: copyediting and, 62; duplication and, 32, 193, 199; ethics and, 32, 62, 166, 192–93, 199; non-native users of English and, 166; permissions and, 32; software for detecting, 32
Plain Language Thesaurus for Health Communications (CDC), 163
plainlanguage.gov, 30
plurals, 16, 70, 92
points of entry, 164
poster presentations, 142–45, 158
PowerPoint, 31
prepositions, 69, 162, 167–68, 185
preprint server, 44
preprints, 16, 44
press releases. *See* news releases
pre-submission editing, 50, 55
principal investigators (PIs), 45, 72, 134, 200, 248
Principles of Scientific Writing and Biomedical Publication (Fontanarosa, Flanagin, and Greenland), 21
PRISMA (**P**referred **R**eporting **I**tems for **S**ystematic reviews and **M**eta-**A**nalyses), 122
proceedings, 139, 145–48, 158, 240
production editors, 5, 8, 41, 46, 204
professional references, 214
pronouns, 70, 79, 83, 172
proofreading: *AMA Manual of Style* and, 171; AMWA and, 51, 172; author's editors and, 170; capitalization and, 185; captions and, 171; careers and, 209, 213, 219; Chartered Institute of Editing and Proofreading, 27; clarity and, 171; commas and, 170, 172; comparison, 172; conciseness and, 159–62; conferences and, 148; consistency and, 172; content and, 172; copyediting and, 88; corrections and, 51, 170–71; cover letters and, 209; dead copy, 172; format and, 171; freelancers and, 172; grammar and, 170–71; grant proposals and, 171; journal articles and, 170; live copy, 172; manuscripts

and, 170–72; mechanical errors and, 170, 185; non-comparison, 172; orphans and, 171; PDF files and, 171; PerfectIt, 32; pre-submission, 44, 51; publishers and, 171–72; punctuation and, 170, 172; resources for, 27, 32, 170–72; role of, 5, 170–72, 185; serial comma and, 170; spelling and, 19, 32, 70, 85, 154, 170, 172; style and, 170–72; submission and, 170–72; Track Changes and, 171; typographical errors and, 51, 98, 170–72, 185; verbs and, 185; widows and, 170–71

proofs: accuracy and, 41; conferences and, 148; reviewing, 41, 44, 51, 148, 170–72

public information officer, 126

publication: author relationships and, 180–81; careers and, 203–4, 221, 224, 230; conferences and, 139; copyediting and, 43, 59–60, 65, 67, 76, 88; ethics and, 180, 187, 190–99; exercises and, 246; resources for, 14, 16–17, 23–24, 29–31; role of, 4–7; style and, 7, 13–18, 22, 25, 43, 51, 59–60, 65, 67, 76, 84–88, 92, 170, 196; substantive editing and, 106, 112–13, 124

publication editing, 55–56

publication histories, 29, 155

publication lists, 155–57

Publication Manual of the American Psychological Association (American Psychological Association), 14, 76

publicity, 41

publishers: book proposals and, 46; careers and, 229–31; conferences and, 147; copyediting and, 68, 75; ethics and, 196; format and, 2, 6, 14, 22, 51, 171; proofreading and, 171–72; resources for, 14, 17, 22, 28; role of, 2, 6, 8, 11; substantive editing and, 96

PubMed, 29, 35, 100, 103

pull quotes, 164

punctuation: colons, 67, 101, 236; compound sentences, 65; copyediting and, 59, 64–70, 85–87, 90, 92; em dashes, 67; en dashes, 67; mechanical errors and, 64–70, 85–87, 90, 92; non-native users of English and, 168; pitfalls and, 174; proofreading and, 170, 172; quotation marks, 85, 239; resources for, 14–15, 19, 27, 30; role of, 1, 5, 9; semicolons, 66–67; serial comma, 14, 17–18, 51, 53, 85, 88, 125, 156, 170, 229, 236, 239; style sheets and, 236, 239; substantive editing and, 95; verbs and, 236

Purdue University Online Writing Lab (OWL), 14, 30

QR (quick response) codes, 145

queries: author relationships and, 60–64, 176–81, 184; careers and, 149–50, 218–19; commissioning editors and, 181, 184; conciseness and, 161–62; copyediting and, 58–64, 80–82, 89–91; corrections and, 60–61; ethics and, 191, 199; non-native users of English and, 167; numbers and, 62; pitfalls and, 175; resources for, 33; role of, 10; substantive editing and, 97, 99, 103–9, 114, 128; Track Changes and, 61–64

query letter (pitch), 47, 181

quizzes, 16, 20, 64, 89

quotation marks, 85, 239

Radiological Society of North America, 28

rationality, 188, 198
readability: ambiguity and, 44, 48, 68, 82, 152, 174, 206; application essays and, 154; conciseness and, 184; content and, 162–63; deck and, 164; format and, 164; general readership and, 163–64; *Guidelines for Document Designers* and, 163; logic and, 164; magazines and, 164; points of entry, 164; pull quotes and, 164; resources for, 163; sidebars and, 164; statistics and, 164; websites and, 163. *See also* clarity
recommendation letters, 21, 149–51, 158
Recommendations for Promoting Integrity in Scientific Journal Publications (Council of Science Editors Editorial Policy Committee), 22, 194, 196–97
"Recommendations for the Conduct, Reporting, Editing, and Publication of Scholarly Work in Medical Journals" (ICMJE), 196–97
RefWorks, 33
Regulatory Affairs Professionals Society (RAPS), 21, 23, 25
Regulatory Writing (DeTora), 21
rejection, 39–43, 50, 181
resources: abbreviations, 14–15, 19; acronyms, 19; AI, 33, 227; AMWA, 19, 23–24, 26, 33, 51; AP style, 14, 18; APA style, 17–18; author relationships, 184; Board of Editors in the Life Sciences, 24; capitalization, 15–16, 19; career, 203–5, 209–10, 215, 219–28; case reports, 21; certificates, 19, 22, 24–26, 35; certification, 24, 31; conferences, 16, 22–24, 33, 142, 146; consistency, 19; content, 15, 17–20, 23–24, 30; COPE, 30, 196–97; copyediting, 16, 19–20, 31, 34, 60, 76, 87, 91, 184; copyeditors, 19–20, 34; CSE, 13–14, 17–18, 22–24, 33; degrees, 26–27, 32, 35; dictionaries, 18–19, 28–29, 34; drugs, 29; EASE, 23–24; Editorial Freelancers Association, 24, 223–24; educational, 13, 16, 19, 24–28, 31, 35; email discussion lists, 22, 24–25, 31, 34, 175, 197, 224, 227; EQUATOR, 30; ethics, 14–16, 19, 22, 30, 189–97; format, 14, 22, 33; freelancers, 21–24, 27, 31, 34, 223–24; general readership, 14, 18, 21, 24, 29–30; grammar, 15–16, 19, 27, 30, 32, 154, 168; grant proposals, 21, 23, 26–27; hyphens, 16, 19, 24; instructions to authors, 30, 34; *JAMA*, 28–29, 155; magazines, 26; manuscripts, 15–23, 29–33; mentors, 11, 22, 25; news releases, 14, 18; news stories, 18; NIH, 29, 32, 44–45; non-native users of English, 169; nouns, 32; numerical, 14–15, 17; online forums, 22, 31, 34, 175, 197, 224, 227; PDF files, 32; peer review, 23; pitfalls, 173, 175; preprints, 16; professional organizations, 13, 22–25, 31, 35; proofreading, 27, 32, 170–72; publication, 14, 16–17, 23–24, 29–31; publishers, 14, 17, 22, 28; punctuation, 14–15, 19, 27, 30; queries, 33; readability, 163; respect, 34; review articles, 16, 21, 29; revisions, 21; science writing, 23–24, 26, 184; scientific editors, 22–24; scientific papers, 21, 23; scientific writing, 20, 26, 30; spelling, 18–19, 29; statistical, 15, 19, 21, 27, 32; style manuals, 13–18, 20, 22, 28, 34, 51, 55, 63–64, 67, 70–71, 75–82, 85–90, 147,

170–72, 181, 194–97, 217, 236; substantive editing, 137, 164; verbs, 32; websites, 14, 16–17, 19, 22–26, 30–31; word usage, 15. *See also* online resources; *and specific publications*
respect: author relationships and, 176; copyediting and, 76–79, 92; courtesy and, 9–10, 12; ethics and, 188, 198; non-native users of English and, 165; resources for, 34; wording and, 76–79, 92
resumes: biosketches and, 155–58; careers and, 149, 155–58, 212–14, 231; preparation of, 212–14. *See also* curriculum vitae (CVs)
Retraction Watch, 196–97
review articles: classification of, 117; IMRAD format and, 116, 118; resources for, 16, 21, 29; substantive editing and, 100, 116–18, 122, 135
revisions: acceptance and, 43; author relationships and, 176–83; bias and, 76–79; conferences and, 141, 146–48; copyediting and, 59–61, 82–83; corrections and, 52–53, 60; ethics and, 191; exercises and, 242; journal articles and, 37, 40–41, 101; non-native users of English and, 166; resources for, 21; substantive editing and, 99, 101, 104, 109, 113, 118, 127, 136
Rising Scholars, 27, 228
rough drafts, 49
running titles, 102

salami science (cucumber science), 193, 199
Saller, Carol Fisher, 20, 173
Science Editor (journal), 22, 184, 193, 224
science writing: careers and, 210; National Association of Science Writers, 23–24, 184, 228; resources for, 23–24, 26, 184; substantive editing and, 123
scientific editors: resources for, 22–24; role of, 4. *See also* Council of Science Editors (CSE)
Scientific Editors Network (ScENe), 24
scientific papers: author relationships and, 176, 180; careers and, 151, 156; conciseness and, 162; conferences and, 143; copyediting and, 74; ethics and, 196; resources for, 21, 23; role of, 4; substantive editing and, 99–100, 109, 113, 116, 118, 122–23
scientific writing, 20, 26, 30, 168
screening, 39–42, 46, 136, 208–9, 242
semicolons, 66–67
sentence structure, 19, 151, 161, 168, 173–74, 185
serial commas: copyediting and, 85, 88; proofreading and, 170; style and, 14, 17–18, 51, 53, 85, 88, 125, 156, 170, 229, 236, 239; substantive editing and, 125
side effects, 67, 101, 110, 126
sidebars, 164
slide presentations, 140–42, 158
spacing, 51, 57, 87, 157, 168, 170–71
specialists: careers and, 150; conferences and, 146; copyediting and, 83; role of, 6; substantive editing and, 119
specific aims, 130–31
spellcheckers, 19, 32, 70, 85, 154
spelling: copyediting and, 60–64, 70–73, 79, 85, 90, 92; correcting, 5, 9, 29, 53, 60–61, 95, 170; preferred, 85–86; proofreading and, 170, 172; resources for, 18–19, 29; style sheets and, 240; substantive editing and, 95

stacked nouns, 84
statement of purpose, 151, 157
statistics: copyediting and, 64, 79–82, 92; exercises and, 244; readability and, 164; resources for, 15, 19, 21, 27, 32; style and, 15, 82; substantive editing and, 81–82, 103, 106–9, 112–13, 131, 137
Stedman's Medical Dictionary, 18–19, 32
STROBE (**ST**rengthening the **R**eporting of **OB**servational studies in **E**pidemiology), 123
structured abstracts, 103–4, 115
study sections, 45
style: author relationships and, 181–82; careers and, 156, 158, 213–14, 217, 225; citation, 86, 147, 192; conferences and, 140, 146–48; conformity to, 84–88; context, 18, 55, 71, 84, 116; copyediting and, 59–67, 70–92; ethics and, 192–97, 201; exercises and, 241, 250; figures, 87–88; format, 1–2, 6–7, 14, 22, 41, 43, 51, 55, 59–61, 71, 75, 86–88, 92, 116, 121, 124–25, 146–47, 156, 170, 196; grant proposals, 67, 75, 96, 134; manuals, 13–22, 28, 34, 51, 55, 63–64, 67, 70–71, 75–82, 85–90, 147, 170–72, 181, 194–97, 217, 236; mechanical errors and, 51, 53–54, 60, 65, 170, 201, 250; medical editing sense, 84–87; nomenclature, 10, 14–15, 18, 74–75; non-native users of English and, 169; numbers, 86; pitfalls and, 174; proofreading and, 170–72; publication, 7, 13–18, 22, 25, 43, 51, 59–60, 65, 67, 76, 84–88, 92, 170, 196; required, 1–2, 6–7, 43, 50, 53, 71, 77, 87–88, 90, 99; resources for, 13–22, 25, 27–28, 31, 34; role of, 1–2, 6–7; spacing and, 51, 57, 87, 157, 168, 170–71; statistics and, 15, 82; submission and, 7, 50–51, 96; substantive editing and, 96, 99, 116, 121, 124–26, 129, 134; tables and, 87–88
style sheets: abstracts and, 235–38; acronyms and, 237, 240; *AMA Manual of Style* and, 27; capitalization and, 237; careers and, 158; conferences and, 147–48; copyediting and, 87–88; copyeditors and, 236, 239; as crucial tool, 87–88, 92; dictionaries and, 147, 236, 239; general readers and, 239–40; hyphens and, 237; importance of, 87–88; instructions to authors and, 236; journal articles and, 235; manuscript editors and, 235; numbers and, 236–37, 239; proceedings and, 240; proofreading and, 170; punctuation and, 236, 239; spelling and, 240; substantive editing and, 99; verbs and, 236
subject-verb agreement, 51, 68–69
submission: author relationships and, 177, 179, 182; author's editors and, 8, 39; careers and, 204–5; conferences and, 146; copyediting and, 90, 96, 103, 112, 116, 134; ethics and, 192–95; exercises and, 249; journal articles and, 4–5, 8, 39, 43–44, 50, 90, 96, 103, 116, 170, 172, 179, 192–95, 204–5; presubmission editing and, 50, 55; proofreading and, 170–72; style and, 7, 50–51, 96
substantive editing: abbreviations and, 104, 133; abstracts and, 99, 101, 103–5, 115, 117–19, 122, 130, 137; acronyms and, 122, 133; *AMA Manual of Style* and, 125; AP style and, 124; authorship and, 102–3, 112, 115; captions and, 129;

careers and, 149–53, 204, 219, 229; case reports and, 95–97, 116, 118–22, 135; clarity and, 104, 112, 127, 133, 135; completeness and, 96–97, 135; conciseness and, 104, 127; conferences and, 139, 146; conflicts of interest and, 96, 126; consistency and, 99, 101, 107, 132–34; CONSORT and, 101, 122; content and, 95–104, 107–9, 115–17, 121–22, 125–29, 132–37; context and, 101, 104–5, 109–11, 114–16, 119–22, 126, 130, 135, 137; contributors and, 102–3, 134; copyediting and, 61, 81, 91, 95–96, 99, 113, 120–21, 130, 159; drugs and, 101, 107, 119, 125, 250; education and, 98, 119, 123, 130, 134; EQUATOR and, 121–23, 135; ethics and, 96, 98, 127, 135; feature articles and, 127–29; feedback and, 112, 137–38; focus and, 96–97, 101, 109–12, 117–20, 126–30, 133, 135; format and, 99, 101, 103–4, 109, 114–18, 121, 124–27, 132, 135; freelancers and, 96, 123, 130; funding sources and, 113, 115, 130–32; general readership and, 123–29, 135; grammar and, 95, 127; grant proposals and, 95–96, 130–35; IMRAD and, 99–103, 114–18, 121, 135; indexes and, 105; instructions to authors and, 105; integrity and, 102; inverted pyramid format, 124–25, 127; journal articles and, 95–96, 99–127, 133–37; keywords and, 103–5, 127; logic and, 1, 96–98, 106, 111, 117, 135; magazines and, 123–24; manuscripts and, 96, 99–100, 103, 106, 109–14; news releases and, 123–29, 135; news stories and, 123–29; non-native users of English and, 165; nursing journals and, 105; organization and, 95–97, 108, 132, 134–37; peer review and, 99, 111, 130–31; permissions and, 98, 119; PRISMA and, 122; public information officers and, 126; publication and, 106, 112–13, 124; publishers and, 96; punctuation and, 95; queries and, 97, 99, 103–9, 114, 128; rationale for, 96–99; resources for, 164; review articles and, 100, 116–18, 122, 135; revisions and, 99, 101, 104, 109, 113, 118, 127, 136; role of, 96–99; running titles and, 102; science writing and, 123; scientific papers and, 99–100, 109, 113, 116, 118, 122–23; scope of, 96–99; serial commas and, 125; specialists and, 119; spelling and, 95; statistics and, 81–82, 103, 106–9, 112–13, 131, 137; structured abstracts and, 103–4, 115; style and, 96, 99, 116, 121, 124–26, 129, 134; summary leads and, 124; websites and, 121–24, 135

Subversive Copy Editor, The (Saller), 20, 173

summary leads, 124

syntax, 82–84, 220

tables, 88–91

tagging, 91

technical editors, 208

technical reports, 6

tests, 217–18, 235–36

Texas A&M University Writing Center, 30

Text Recycling Research Project, 193

toponyms, 75–76

Track Changes: author relationships and, 179, 181; copyediting and, 60–61; explanations and, 52, 55; No Markup setting, 57; proofreading and, 171; queries and, 61–64; Word and, 31

tracking of paper, 40
transparency: EQUATOR and, 30, 121–23, 135; ethics and, 111, 188, 190, 198, 245; substantive editing and, 111, 113, 121–23, 135
trustworthiness, 188, 198
tweets, 6
typographical errors, 51, 98, 170–72, 185

unbiased wording, 6, 10, 76–79, 92, 190
universalizability, 188, 198
University of California, San Diego, 26
University of Chicago, 26
University of Chicago Press, 14, 20, 51, 76, 171
University of Texas MD Anderson Cancer Center, 28, 61, 184
University of Toledo, 30
URL (uniform resource locator), 28, 72
US Government Printing Office, 14
US Public Health Service, 59
USAJOBS, 208

veracity, 187, 198
verbs: conciseness and, 160–61, 184; grammar and, 32, 51, 66, 68–69, 160–61, 168, 184–85, 236; non-native users of English and, 168; nouns derived from, 160–61; proofreading and, 185; punctuation and, 236; resources for, 32; singular, 66; style sheets and, 236; subject agreement and, 51, 68–69; tenses of, 168
visibility, 31, 49, 57, 171

webinars, 22–23, 25, 33, 172, 226–28
websites: author relationships and, 177, 179, 181, 251; careers and, 155, 157, 205, 208, 215, 222–24, 231; conferences and, 141; copyediting and, 86, 89; ethics and, 194, 196; non-native users of English and, 169; readability and, 163; resources for editors, 14, 16–17, 19, 22–26, 30–31; substantive editing and, 121–24, 135
What to Charge (Lewis), 22, 223
widows, 170–71
word usage: commonly confused terms, 73–74; copyediting and, 59, 64, 73–76, 92; corrections and, 5, 9; nomenclature and, 74–75; resources for, 15; respectful, 76–79; unbiased, 76–79
World Association of Medical Editors (WAME), 23
World Health Organization (WHO), 8, 76
"Writing for the World" (Walshe, Beernart, Chong, et al.), 169

Zeiger, Mimi, 21
Zoom, 167, 215, 224
Zotero, 33